Praise for Dr. Jeffry S. Life and **THE LIFE PLAN**

"Having known Dr. Life for over a decade I've been continually inspired by his ongoing transformation. He's showing that remarkable physical fitness and vitality can be achieved at any age. He is a true expert who has the unique combination of a physician's intellect and the practical wisdom which can only be achieved when you combine knowing what to do with doing what you know. Long live life!"

—Bill Phillips, #1 *New York Times* bestselling author of
Body-for-LIFE and founder of Transformation.com

"Dr. Life's book is life-changing . . . a fabulous read."

—Suzanne Somers, #1 *New York Times*
bestselling author of *Sexy Forever*

"Since I've been under the care of Dr. Life, my goal of living a productive life until at least 100 seems possible. My overall health has improved dramatically and I look and feel many years younger. I've recommended Dr. Life to all of my friends."

—Rick Barry, member of the Basketball Hall of
Fame and an NBA All-Time Top 50 Player

"Exercise and nutrition are the paths to feeling and looking good. Dr. Life's book explains his methods in easy-to-understand terms, and his physique and mind proves that it works."

—Lawrence A. Golding, Ph.D., FACSM, exercise
physiologist, University of Nevada, Las Vegas

"Read on and change your life."

—Steve Miller, former NFL football player and former
director of Global Sports Marketing, Nike, Inc.

"Achieving and maintaining balance is the primary goal in my life. That is why I follow the expertise of Dr. Life."

—Cesar Millan, TV star and dog behaviorist

THE LIFE PLAN

How Any Man Can Achieve Lasting Health,
Great Sex, and a Stronger, Leaner Body

Jeffry S. Life, M.D., Ph.D.

ATRIA PAPERBACK

New York   London   Toronto   Sydney   New Delhi

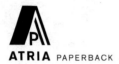

ATRIA PAPERBACK

A Division of Simon & Schuster, Inc.
1230 Avenue of the Americas
New York, NY 10020

First Atria Paperback edition July 2012

ATRIA PAPERBACK and colophon are trademarks of Simon & Schuster, Inc.

For information about special discounts for bulk purchases, please contact Simon & Schuster Special Sales at 1-866-506-1949 or business@simonandschuster.com.

The Simon & Schuster Speakers Bureau can bring authors to your live event. For more information or to book an event, contact the Simon & Schuster Bureau at 1-866-248-3049 or visit our website at www.simonspeakers.com.

Designed by Jason Snyder

Manufactured in the United States of America

10   9   8   7   6   5   4   3   2

Library of Congress Cataloging-in-Publication Data

Life, Jeffry S.
   The life plan: Dr. Life's guide for men to great health, better sex, and a stronger, leaner body/Jeffry S. Life.
      p. cm.
   Includes bibliographical references and index.
   1. Men—Health and hygiene. I. Title.
   RA777.8.L54 2011
   613'.0423—dc22

                                          2010041265

ISBN 978-1-4391-9458-4
ISBN 978-1-4391-9459-1 (pbk)
ISBN 978-1-4391-9460-7 (ebook)

This book is dedicated to my dear friend Alan P. Mintz, M.D.,
(May 5, 1938–June 3, 2007),
"The Father of Age Management Medicine,"
whose wisdom and vision inspired me to create this book.

Contents

THE
LIFE
PLAN

Introduction

Most men, including myself, define themselves in two distinct ways: by what we do for a living and by how things are going in bed. If either one goes awry, we instantly feel less "manly." That's true whether you're 25 or 80. We need to know that we can still compete, that we are still in the game, and that there's much more to look forward to even as we approach or pass midlife.

Yet men don't realize that both of these barometers are directly connected to their health. When we feel healthy, vibrant, and young, we excel in the workplace and can keep up with our sexual instincts. But when our health begins to decline, everything about life suffers. That's why I recommend a proactive approach to health, which is exactly what age management medicine is all about. Sitting back, not taking control of your health, and simply accepting the status quo is a guarantee that you'll age faster and be at much greater risk for disease. Healthy aging begins by taking care of yourself now, so that you don't pay for it later when chronic disease rears its ugly head and "surprises" you. Take it from me: When I was in my 20s and 30s, I was already developing heart disease without even knowing it. And by the time I woke up to this realization, I had wasted many decades of good health and had to work very hard to get it back.

My Story

Regardless of whether I'm speaking with the media or a new patient, the first questions anyone ever asks me are always: "Are your photos real?" "How did this happen? How did you turn a 50-something potbellied body into a healthy, 30-something physique?" I'm not offended or embarrassed: With our programmed view of aging—and our overexposure to airbrushed tabloid photos—it's easy to understand the doubt. A 72-year-old with a strong physique, low body fat, lots of lean muscle mass, and optimized health goes entirely against conventional thinking.

I'm also not embarrassed to say that I could have easily continued my life the way it was and completely missed the boat to great health. And that's why my story is so important for every man to hear, because I was you, and I know how to change the way you age because I have done it and am continuing to do it today.

In 1994, I was going through a divorce and had reached an all-time low in terms of my self-esteem, mood, level of fitness, and appearance. I had been working in my family medical practice for 16 years, treating people of all ages from all walks of life. Even though my business was thriving, I had really lost enthusiasm for my work. I was living under a dark cloud, but there was a silver lining. In December of that year I met the love of my life, Annie. Over the next few years Annie and I were together constantly. I was happy most of the time, yet I continued to struggle with poor self-esteem, lousy fitness, and excess body fat.

Then in 1998, I came to the frightening realization that I looked and felt like an old man. My joints and muscles ached, I had shortness of breath whenever I climbed just one flight of stairs, my clothes were tight, and my stomach was huge. My LDL (bad cholesterol) scores were sky-high, my HDL (good cholesterol) numbers were rock bottom, and I was well on my way to becoming a full-blown type 2 diabetic. At 59 years old I was already a senior citizen with a pot belly, fatigue, sluggish thinking, out-of-control blood sugar, and undiagnosed heart disease. My self-esteem had never been lower and my waist never bigger. I, like most men my age, had devoted my time and energy to my career and family, which meant putting myself dead last.

On top of all this, my sex life was in trouble. My interest in sex was almost nonexistent. I suffered from erectile dysfunction, which, coupled with my low self-esteem, led to a daily battle with anxiety and depression. The irony, of course, was that I am a physician certified in family medicine who should know about staying fit and eating right. But that's exactly what the issue was: I didn't know. Like most in my profession, I had no nutritional or exercise training, and I knew nothing about the importance of hormone therapies and their relationship to healthy aging. As a result, I had become just another middle-aged man, the byproduct of conventional medical thinking and a disease-oriented approach to health—trained to ignore the hope that my life could get better instead of worse as I got older.

Then, one day, I took a long, hard look in the mirror. What I saw made me realize if I didn't begin focusing on my own health, there would be no future. I knew I had to change my life drastically if I was going to maintain an active relationship with my kids, grandkids, and my beautiful girlfriend (now wife), who was almost 20 years younger than me.

Around that same time, someone had given me an issue of *Muscle Media*, a magazine written and published by Bill Phillips, owner of EAS Corporation. I took it home that night and read it cover to cover. I signed up that night for a lifetime subscription.

Soon after that, I ran into Pat Graham, an old nursing colleague from the emergency department where I had worked a couple of years before. Pat looked great: She had lost several pounds and was super fit. I asked her how she had been able to achieve her new physique, and she told me about her personal trainer, Ernie. Ernie owned a gym not far from me, so I decided to go check him out. When I walked into his gym I was met by a 50-year-old muscular Marine-looking guy behind the counter. I told him that he had been recommended to me as a guy who could really help me get in shape. He looked me up and down and said, "I don't know, old man. That looks like quite a challenge."

This was the beginning of a love-hate relationship between me and a Navy SEAL who had fought two tours of duty in Vietnam, then incorporated all he learned into physical fitness training. One month into his balls-to-the-wall program I read about the first winners of the 1997 Body-*for*-LIFE contest. I looked at the before-and-after pictures and thought to myself, *These people can't be for real.* I was amazed at the way so many people had transformed themselves, over such a short period of time, from being fat and out of shape to being fit and lean. If those contestants could transform their bodies, maybe I could, too. I showed the pictures to Annie, and she immediately said I should enter the 1998 contest.

I raced to have my "before" pictures taken, then hired Keith Klein, a bodybuilder/nutritionist from Texas, and I started my pursuit of Bill Phillips's challenge. I told Ernie what I wanted to do and he said, "Okay, old man, but we better step up your program." I had just 19 weeks to make a significant change in every aspect of my life. Instead of drinking often and eating poorly, I put myself on a low-glycemic/low-fat diet, took supplements, stayed away from alcohol, and plunged into an exercise program.

Quite honestly, the first few weeks were pretty rough: I felt sore and beat up most of the time. I had been training three times a week with Ernie, and now we increased the schedule to five times a week. He said, "Old man, I doubt that you are going to be able to train as hard as you need to win this contest, but we are going to go for it." So five mornings a week, I would get up at 4:00 A.M. and drive to Ernie's gym. I had to train very early in the morning so I could make it to my office by nine o'clock. Ernie pushed me to limits I had never dreamed possible.

He lived by the "no-pain-no-gain" principle. He taught me how to lift weights, how to build muscle and strength, how to eat clean, and how to lose body fat. More important, he helped me reach down deep into myself and maximize every last bit of my potential. He gave me the desire to set goals as high as possible and gave me the tools to reach those goals in small, precise steps. Ernie changed the way I think about myself.

Gradually I began to see real results. My LDL (bad cholesterol) went from 164 down to 80, and I started feeling better and stronger. What's more, I could see the change in my physique. I was beginning to like the guy in the mirror. I also became extremely interested in nutrition and, thanks to a suggestion from a nutritionist at my office, I checked out a master's degree in sports nutrition at Marywood University in Scranton, Pennsylvania. Not long after, I was accepted into the program and started classes with the 20-year-olds while continuing to practice family medicine full-time and preparing for the Body-*for*-LIFE challenge.

By the end of 1998, at age 60, I had my after pictures taken and then submitted an essay about how the Body-*for*-LIFE program had helped me. A week or so later, Bill Phillips's mother called me and told me I was one of the finalists in my age category. Then, on Monday, December 7, I got a call from Porter Freeman, the 1997 winner in my age category and the new director of the program. Porter immediately asked me, "What would you do, Dr. Life, if you were the winner?" I thought he was just jerking me around until he told me the real news: I *was* the winner.

I hung up and still didn't believe it. I sat there for a few minutes, and then suddenly the phone rang. It was Amy, Bill's assistant. She said, "I am calling you so I can make arrangements for you to fly out to Denver."

After just 19 weeks of eating and training right, I had become a Grand Champion in Bill Phillips's 1998 Body-*for*-LIFE contest. The sense of accomplishment was overwhelming. Bill knew I had gone back to school to study nutrition and exercise science, and he came up to me during the awards dinner and asked me to be a contributing writer for *Muscle Media* magazine. I wrote a monthly column titled Ask Dr. Life, which I happily did for the next four years. This marked the beginning of my writing career.

After winning the Body-*for*-LIFE contest I immediately started incorporating my new lifestyle into my medical practice. Previously, I had doctored my patients the same way most physicians did: Almost all the care I provided centered on treating existing disease. But once I realized how much better I felt when I took a proactive approach, I began to change my focus to disease prevention and attempted to get my patients to start improving their health through better eating and exercise. It was truly an uphill battle, but I persevered. My patient population was typical of most Americans: They just did not want to do much in terms of improving their health and well-being.

I continued to train consistently and ate pretty clean. But a few years later, I began to notice that I was losing ground—gaining abdominal fat and losing muscle mass as well as strength, plus my energy and sexual function were also taking a hit. It was frustrating, to say the least. I knew I had a predisposition toward diabetes and heart disease because of my family history, but my regimen hadn't changed: I was training as hard as ever with Ernie, but not seeing the same results. I was actually getting worse.

I realized that everything was becoming more difficult, whether it was getting up and practicing medicine, going to the gym, or making love with my wife. Then, in 2003, I came across a brochure for a medical meeting in Las Vegas regarding the role nutrition plays in preventing disease. The sponsor of the meeting was Barry Sears of Zone Diet fame. I signed up and headed out to Las Vegas. I met several Cenegenics Medical Institute doctors, as well as Dr. Alan Mintz and John Adams, the founders of this national medical practice. I learned then that they promoted an exercise and nutrition program in combination with correcting hormonal deficiencies, an entirely new concept for me. I signed up that day for the Cenegenics physician training program in age management medicine. The soonest opening available was going to be in August.

I went back to Pennsylvania and began wondering about my own hormone levels. I decided to get my levels checked at my local lab and learned I had major deficiencies in testosterone, DHEA, and growth hormone. That explained my losing muscle mass, strength, and endurance—and why I also was accumulating body fat and battling low energy levels, sluggish thinking, and even depression. I knew I had been getting viral infections more often, but guessed it was due to the fact that as a doctor I was constantly exposed to illnesses. But in reality, my immune system had significantly declined. The diminished hormones also explained the other major wall I had hit: a decrease in sexual function.

Enough was enough. I called John Adams and asked if there was any way I could start my age management program before I came out in August for my training. John was able to find a specialist to work with me. I became a patient of Cenegenics in June 2003.

Two months later, when I flew to Las Vegas to meet with John and Alan and begin my professional Cenegenics training, I had already noticed profound changes in my physique and energy levels. My physician had corrected my hormone deficiencies and had me continue a low-glycemic/low-fat nutrition program, the right exercise, and key supplements. I went from exhausted to exhilarated as I started getting my strength back. Once again I was losing body fat and gaining clarity in my thinking, and my sexual function came back as well. Cenegenics had helped me regain what Bill Phillips had given me—and what aging was taking away from me.

John, Alan, and the staff were very impressed with me and what I had accomplished. On day two of my training, they offered me a job. In January 2004, I became a Senior Institute Physician for Cenegenics and moved out to Las Vegas.

Six years after I won the Body-for-LIFE contest, I decided to get some pictures taken of myself without a shirt to show my patients I still was living the lifestyle I was preaching. In late 2005, a freelance writer was doing a story for *GQ* magazine on Cenegenics. When he was interviewing me, he noticed my picture on the wall and asked if he could use it in the article.

In early 2006, the article came out in *GQ*, and I was inundated by hundreds of phone calls. Not long after that, the Cenegenics marketing firm thought it would be a good idea to use my picture in one of its ads. Later my wife, Annie, got the idea of placing it in *US Airways* magazine to help me promote my own practice at Cenegenics. This proved to be a very successful marketing strategy. To this day Cenegenics continues to use my image in the majority of its marketing materials and campaigns.

It has now been 13 years since I began this journey. What's so exciting to me is that not only do I feel great, I've been able to actually improve my physique over the years. I have been able to stay lean, reduce my cholesterol levels, reduce internal or "silent" inflammation, reduce blood sugar levels, and avoid diabetes. I have stopped the progression of heart disease that started when I was in my 20s. I have mental focus, clarity, and sharpness like I never had before. I am more productive and creative than ever, and I'm stronger and have more muscle mass than ever. At 72, I love being married to Annie, building my medical practice and website, writing my book, training for my black belt in martial arts, riding my Harley, playing with my grandkids, and learning more about exercise, nutrition, and preventive medicine. I love being energetic, lean, fit, and muscular. I love training with people half my age and continuing my education surrounded by 20-year-olds. In the summer of 2013, I will have earned my executive MBA degree from Auburn University.

My cardiologist and I both strongly believe that had I not entered into this journey back in 1998, I would not be here today. For that reason alone, my mission is to share this new paradigm with as many people as possible. Helping men take charge of their health and work proactively toward their goals, not to mention witnessing their own transformations, is hugely satisfying both personally and professionally.

Now it's your turn. I have taken everything I've learned on this journey and put it into this book so you can begin yours.

What Aging Really Means

To me, the very word "aging" conjures up certain images: an old man who has no sex life, no physical energy, a flabby body, no muscle tone, weakness, slowed thinking, fragile bones, stooped posture, debilitating disease, hospital stays, nursing homes—basically, an end to life. You might already be experiencing some of these signs and symptoms. Your doctor may notice them as well, but is probably writing them off as "typical aging." Stop right there. You don't have to accept that aging is synonymous with declining health, or that becoming a shadow of your former self is a reluctant rite of passage. I'm here to tell you that as you age, you don't have to get old. Instead, you can get better. Don't just take my word for it: Study after study shows that the right lifestyle interventions can eliminate, prevent, delay, or even reverse aging and age-related diseases. But you have to know the rules and the secrets of healthy living. That's what this book is all about.

I was once taking a walk with my then 70-year-old father, who had retired to Florida. He was just poking along and finally said, "Jeff, you've got to slow down." It surprised me because I was walking at a leisurely pace. He would become short of breath—and not because of a heart condition or obesity, but because he was deconditioned. He actually thought that deconditioning was an inevitable part of the aging process, so he reluctantly accepted it.

Even then I realized I couldn't accept aging if that was what it meant for me. My dad never got his heart rate up above 80: Exercise just wasn't part of his life. No wonder his body was stiff and slowing down to where he couldn't even enjoy a casual walk.

In all fairness, his attitude was typical of his generation. Exercise, for all intents and purposes, was to be avoided. Retirement was all about not working, and this meant doing next to nothing. When my father retired at 65, he sat in his La-Z-Boy most of the day. He may have lived to his 80s, but certainly not with the quality of life he could have had.

Studies over the past decade have shown that the "old man" excuses are way off. We may inherit genetic potential, but we definitely don't inherit genetic certainty. Lifestyle changes—like the ones I'll share with you—can dramatically reduce your mortality risk and slow your aging process. You can get better as you get older. I turned 72 in 2010, but my body looks and feels much younger. My energy levels are every bit as good as when I was in my 30s and are actually, in many ways, better. I'm not telling you this to brag, I'm telling you this to get you to change the way you think about aging.

Now, I can't promise you'll live longer, but you'll certainly add a lot more life to the days, weeks, and years you have ahead. I want the same thing you do—an energized, active lifestyle even into my golden years, not the restricted shadow of a life my father's generation blindly accepted. The best part is that I know we can have it. We now have the knowledge and technology to make it happen. I'm living proof that anybody can follow and succeed with this program.

How This Book Works

My reasons for writing this book are many, but topping the list was a desire to help others get out from underneath America's reactionary approach to medicine—one that negatively affects the aging process—and guide them into a different realm of thinking. What is laid out in this book is a new paradigm, one that defines those later years as robust, embodying the very definition of life: energy, movement, change, adaptation, and growth. It's the same paradigm that works for me and continues to work for my patients. When you follow this program, you will be able to achieve exceptional health, fitness, and vitality, and will see a significant improvement in your sexual function.

Part One helps you identify what your current health status is so you can get right to work. You'll learn how to manage the current medical system so you can get the help you need from your current doctor, or learn what type of doctor you should be seeing—one who understands the importance of preventive care. You'll also jump right into my eating program so you can take your health into your own hands and begin to reverse and eliminate disease right now. This is not your wife's diet, nor your girlfriend's. This diet was created by me, specifically for men.

Part Two outlines my unique exercise program, which incorporates every facet of physical fitness, including cardiovascular workouts, resistance training, balance and stretching exercises, and my favorite, the martial arts. No matter what level of fitness you are currently at—even if you haven't exercised in years—there's an entry place for you to start, and a clearly outlined level of progression. There are also dozens of photographs so that you can follow the directions and watch me complete the exercises so you can make sure that you are using correct form every time. I've also included a method for you to track your progress for the entire Life Plan. Plus, there's expert advice to keep you motivated and silence that nagging voice inside you that insists you can't succeed.

Part Three lets me practice medicine my way: sharing the most recent scientific breakthroughs in age management medicine. You'll learn about the importance of correcting hormone deficiencies, and when it is really necessary. You'll also learn new ways to increase your hormone levels naturally, without medical intervention. I'll teach you about my favorite supplement choices and explain in detail why they are necessary for specific health issues. You'll learn what's on the horizon: the latest science that has clinically shown that we can actually reverse aging on the cellular level. And you'll be able to discuss all of this with your doctor so that you can get the healthcare that you deserve.

Join me on this journey, which is supported by hundreds of peer-reviewed scientific studies. You can become your own health advocate, taking charge of your medical needs and creating lifestyle interventions that will work in a program tailored just for you. I know that if you do, you'll enter a dimension of fitness and well-being you never knew existed. In fact, you should start noticing changes in the first two weeks. All it takes is making up your mind to do it.

It is my hope that this book will help you begin to feel like yourself again. Let's get started.

PART ONE

GET WITH THE LIFE PLAN

CHAPTER 1

Taking Control of Your Health

Every day I witness firsthand how our current medical system creates obstacles that keep men from receiving the best care possible. Instead of preventing disease, traditional medicine can actually interfere with and even delay proper treatment and diagnosis, ultimately lowering the quality of our health. If you let today's medical system make decisions about your health, you have little or no hope of living a higher-quality life with optimized health and reduced risks for disease. Now more than ever you have to take charge of your own health, become better informed, and act as an advocate for your own well-being. These are the tenets of my kind of medicine: where disease prevention based on a treatment paradigm and sustained quality of life are my primary missions.

We are all going to age, but we don't have to get old. Getting old means the deterioration of health, declining energy levels, loss of sexual function, and loss of your zest for life. I don't want any part of that, and I'll bet you don't, either.

When I discovered my own hormone levels were deficient, traditional medical professionals, said that andropause, or declining testosterone, is not a disease, so it shouldn't be treated. They were wrong then, and they're even more wrong now. When I was losing muscle tissue and strength, conventional doctors once again said to just accept that I was getting older, and basically, just get over it. Well, hundreds of my patients, including myself, are proving them wrong every day.

Aging is not the enemy. It's not a disease. In fact, by definition, aging is a gradual change in your body that doesn't result from disease. Disease is the deviation or interruption of the normal function of any part or system of your body. This without doubt includes your endocrine system and the hormones associated with it. Declining hormone levels are the result of a disease process, not aging, and should be treated. In my opinion it's malpractice for doctors to ignore declining hormone levels and write them off as simply an acceptable part of aging. It's just like ignoring high cholesterol levels, high blood pressure, or lung disease caused by cigarette smoking.

Each of us has a unique set of inherited predispositions for certain health issues: That's your DNA code. On top of that, your lifestyle choices contribute to whether these tendencies will materialize. Lifestyle can definitely trump genetics. So instead of accepting a waning sex life or waiting for disease to appear, you can learn how to use my health strategies based on age management medicine to keep your body metabolically and physiologically in balance so you do not get old.

First, let's figure out why you're not in optimal health. The answer for many of us has nothing to do with what you are currently doing. Instead, the problem is the machine we call the American Health Care System.

The Insurance Blockade

You might not realize that for most Americans, the quality of the medical care they receive is determined by men and women they will never meet: those who run the insurance companies. These people decide how often your physician sees you, what medications are prescribed, if diagnostic testing that may signal the onset of a silent disease can be ordered, whether you see a specialist, and when you should be admitted into a hospital. Virtually every medical decision a traditional physician makes today is affected by the insurance industry.

Because of this corporate structure, decision making in the practice of medicine has shifted radically from physicians dedicated to your best interest to organizations bound to financial interests. Most doctors aren't happy with this and find themselves forced into using their medical knowledge and experience for the plan's benefit and economic goals—rather than doing what's best for the patient. Medical services have shifted from the hands of the treating physician to administrators, who in many cases aren't medically trained. Worse, managed care has created an environment in which doctors feel rushed when they see their patients, because more patients per day means more minimum payments from insurers. Their stress becomes your bad service: The patient is left with a ten-minute-or-less office visit with a harried doctor who is focused on managing isolated health problems and dispensing prescriptions. Then, doctors are left to second-guess their findings, which leads you to seek multiple opinions.

Today's physicians are being placed in an uncomfortable position by insurers, which can jeopardize the care they provide to their own patients. Aside from managing your health, your doctor has to control his own costs: This affects his or her decisions about choosing specific medications, determining necessary lab work, doling out a limited number of referrals to specialists, and more. These decisions can directly affect your provider's salary. Economic rationales have now replaced clinical judgment.

According to a study published in the *Commonwealth Fund Quarterly, A Digest of Current Work in Health Policy and Practice,* 56 percent of primary care doctors and 60 percent of specialists in the United States believe their ability to provide quality healthcare has deteriorated over the past ten years. Medicare continues to institute cutbacks for medical services. If all of this isn't bad enough, the number of primary care providers, understandably, has continued to decline year after year. The doctor shortage has reached a catastrophic crisis. Underserved areas in this country currently need almost 17,000 new primary care physicians even before Healthcare Reform is implemented. Our new Healthcare Reform will attempt to reach 30 million new patients needing care.

Worst of all, your healthcare is not keeping up with science. We have just ended a century of unprecedented advances in medical knowledge and technology. Serious medical conditions that were once considered disabling or a death sentence are now curable. Most devastating disease conditions in existence today are now manageable. Yet in spite of all the amazing medical advances in recent years, there exists a great paradox in healthcare today—*we simply cannot afford them!* The economics of today's healthcare has made all of the advances in medical science less and less available—even to those who are willing to pay for them out of pocket. As medical costs continue to soar, patients are increasingly being denied coverage for crucial services by their insurance companies. We have the 37th-worst quality of healthcare in the developed world. Conservative estimates show that over 120,000 Americans die each year from treatable, preventable illnesses that citizens of other countries survive. It doesn't matter whether you are rich, middle class, or poor; insured or uninsured; male or female; young or old. Your health is suffering from the system that is supposed to be managing it.

So what can we do in order to receive the best healthcare possible? The answer is really very simple—don't get sick! We must do everything possible to avoid disease, maintain excellent health, and not get old. Prevention is the answer to America's healthcare crisis. We have the right to know our current health status each and every year, which can be done completely only by proactively screening for silent diseases. Today, these tests are discouraged by insurance carriers who state that these medical tests are "unnecessary." This must change.

The Disease Era Lives On

Nothing the insurance industry can throw at medicine today is worse than the reactionary way doctors are trained to respond to disease. Your physician has to wait for disease to appear and then treat it: a fix-it-when-it's-broken mentality. You literally have to get sick first and hope protocols exist to make you better. But what you may not realize is that an illness begins a cascade of sickness: Once disease sets in it plays havoc on the rest of your body, creating more and more health issues.

It's no wonder the National Center for Health Statistics reports that even while Americans are living longer, they are not necessarily healthier. Population studies by Billy S. Guyton, at the University of Mississippi Medical Center, show we have "increased the length of life, but made no progress in decreasing the length of disability at the end of life." An article in a February 2004 issue of the *American Journal of Medicine* said it's time we abandon a disease-focused medical care approach, which "at best, is out of date and, at worst, harmful."

Meet Richard

A great example of the problem of treating disease instead of preventing it is my patient Richard, a 53-year-old type 2 diabetic who came to my office about a year and a half ago. Richard had a big job, overseeing a large corporation. He was overworked, which left him completely focused on his job and somewhat neglecting his family and his own health. At 5 feet 10 inches and 220 pounds, he already walked and looked like he was in his 60s. He moved slowly and was extremely tired most of the time, and had lost his desire for sex. "I really need help, " he said when he came in. "My doctors aren't really helping me. They only seem concerned about my diabetes. But the rest of my life is falling apart, and my physicians are only concerned with my insulin and blood sugars."

His primary care physician and endocrinologist worked on managing his disease—but I took the proactive approach: completely changing his lifestyle with the goal of eliminating his diabetes. First, I had Richard fill out an extensive questionnaire, and then he took a series of blood tests. Then we talked at length about his life and his lifestyle. He told me he was sleeping in the guest room because his wife couldn't stand his snoring, which would interrupt his sleep and hers, all night long. I quickly realized that beyond the diabetes Richard was also suffering from sleep apnea, which was not diagnosed by his physicians. Before prescribing any medications, I had Richard start my Life Plan, the same one outlined in this book. It consisted of a low-fat/low-glycemic eating plan along with an optimized exercise program that focused on weight training and cardiovascular conditioning. My goal was to get him to shed several pounds and rapidly build muscle mass he had lost over the past 10 to 15 years. Increasing his muscle mass would help improve his metabolism and his ability to control his diabetes. I also wanted to get Richard back into his bedroom, and sleeping with his wife.

Once the blood work came back, I realized I also needed to address his deficient hormone levels and elevated markers of arterial inflammation. I started Richard on a customized nutrition/supplementation and exercise program combined with correction of his hormone deficiencies. The blood test also showed that his diabetes was totally out of control. Hemoglobin A1C is a direct measurement of the amount of sugar that is attached to the hemoglobin molecule and reflects the average blood sugar over a three-month period. Hemoglobin A1Cs in the 6s or above are indicative of diabetes, and his was coming in at 7.3.

Six weeks into the program, Richard came back to my office beaming. He had already lost eight pounds and was on the road to better health. Three months later, his hemoglobin A1C levels dropped to 6. As I continued to fine-tune his hormone levels, improve his nutrition, and increase his exercise regimen, Richard's hemoglobin A1C levels came down to 5.5, clearly in the safe, nondiabetic range. He was 20 pounds lighter, completely off all medication, and had no evidence of any damage to his kidneys, blood vessels, nervous system, and eyes as a result of his diabetes. Everything had been reversed—including his sex life—and his blood vessels were even healthier, proven by carotid ultrasound and endothelial function studies, and a reduction in his markers of vascular inflammation. In his words, "I feel better than I did in my 30s!"

Had Richard not taken a proactive approach and continued with his insurance-based/disease-focused medical care, his story would have had a totally different ending: poorly controlled blood sugar levels, increased body fat, high probability for shortened life span with the full impact of diabetes over the next 5 to 10 years, including impotence, potential blindness, vascular complications, potential amputations, kidney failure, or a heart attack or stroke.

I can't fault his primary care physicians, because they were following the standard "treat the disease after it appears" approach. Doctors are paid to treat—not prevent—disease. The insurance industry does not reward your physician for being proactive about preventing disease. As a matter of fact, your physician is penalized if he or she orders tests not backed up with a disease diagnosis.

The Good Ole American Lifestyle

While uninformed doctors and overall healthcare policies can take some of the rap, we are individuals who operate in the real world of free will. If your health is not perfect, you are not completely without fault or blame. We must all learn how to take responsibility for our own health now, so we can maintain a high quality of life as we age.

Every day the lifestyle choices you make—including the types of foods you eat, the time you put aside to exercise, and the types of exercise you choose—are affecting your health right now, and will affect the way you live in the future. If you're like many Americans, you've shifted from being a couch potato to being a mouse potato, immersed in your computer or favorite electronic gadget. The bottom line is you're still not moving.

Plus, your diet may be filled with processed foods, unhealthy proteins, and simple carbohydrates that accelerate aging and make you old. All of these bad food choices are quickly stored as body fat and arterial plaque, not to mention that they suck the energy right out of you, add weight, and create stroke, diabetes, heart disease, and Alzheimer's disease. Men need to change their ways right now if they want to prevent the accumulation of body fat (or get rid of it if they already have it).

And you must learn how to prevent or reverse the loss of bone and muscle tissue. This becomes critically important as we age if we are to avoid nursing home care, chronic pain, immobilization, mental deterioration, and prescription drug dependency. By adopting health-promoting policies, you can become part of a more "active" aging population who will have:

- Fewer premature deaths in highly productive stages of life

- Fewer disabilities and pain associated with chronic diseases

- More independence and positive life quality

The time to plan and act is now. Remember, we don't die of old age. We die because we allow ourselves to get old. I know that making behavioral changes can be challenging for many reasons, including one I often hear about from patients: money. But the fact is it takes far less to prevent disease than it does to treat it. A study published in *Diabetes Care*, which focused on the costs of a health-promoting diet, indicated that "adopting a diet that more closely follows nutrition recommendations will not increase diet costs." Americans complain about rising prices, but actually we tend to have one of the lowest-priced food supplies globally—and spend the lowest proportion of disposable income on food.

Introducing Age Management Medicine

Fortunately, there is a new medical specialty that deals specifically and exclusively with all of these issues—age management medicine (AMM). Physicians like me who follow this type of medical practice are dedicated to the science of healthy aging. AMM emphasizes the enhancement of health over the treatment of illness, focusing on disease prevention, wellness, and quality of life. These strategies include the intelligent promotion of healthy key hormone levels combined with individualized exercise and nutritional programs specifically designed to lower body fat, increase muscle tissue and strength, reduce risk factors for illness, improve overall cardiovascular fitness, and find and treat asymptomatic vascular disease. I have been practicing age management medicine since I joined Cenegenics in January 2004, and have never looked back. That's because as both a doctor and a patient, I know that my patients and I feel better than we ever have before.

I've learned through my own experience that we must all change our thinking about aging. Older does not mean sicker. The majority of men already possess a genetic makeup that will allow us to live well beyond age 85. The key is to make the best of the genes we have so we can live better, for longer. By incorporating AMM practices into our daily lives we can reverse illness and reduce the time we are sick. We can't stop the aging process, but we can definitely manage it. We can avoid premature disability and death. After all, what are the benefits of living longer if we end up in a nursing home, left with a body or brain that doesn't work?

That's why I'm so very glad you've decided to join me and follow my Life Plan. This book is meant to steer you toward making significant changes to your current behavioral and medical choices. My program is based on the latest science-based protocols that work together with your current lifestyle, making a series of small yet important changes that you can implement right now. As you continue on the program, you will step into new levels of diet and nutrition, as well as new levels of exercise. In many cases, these lifestyle changes will correct any hormone deficiencies you might have by helping you make more of your own hormones. The speed with which you step into this program is entirely up to you, but as you can imagine, the faster you can get to the highest levels of fitness and nutrition, the better the results you'll achieve.

The Life Plan for Better Health

Step One: Recognize the Signs and Symptoms
That Mean "You're Getting Old"

You may have heard of the medical phrase "signs and symptoms." While these words sound innocuous, they really are vital signals to watch for. Signs are literally aspects of your health that your doctor can either see with his or her own eyes or pick up with a diagnostic test. Symptoms are negative experiences that cannot be seen or detected except on your own. Both are critically important to your overall health, because they are a warning of premature aging, illness, and potentially early death.

The following quiz will help you determine if you are currently experiencing either signs or symptoms of aging. Circle T for each true response, and F if this issue never occurs. It doesn't matter what your "score" is at the end of the quiz, because the fix is the same. Even if you have only one "true" response, you may be experiencing a hidden, and often seemingly unrelated illness. For example, erectile dysfunction not only affects your sex life, but could be an early symptom of heart disease. The sooner you can get on the Life Plan and address these issues, the more likely it will be that you can—and should—reverse the damage they have caused.

All of these signs and symptoms should be discussed with your doctor before you begin the program. You'll learn in Chapter 14 exactly how to have this conversation and what your doctor should be doing for you to address these and other health issues.

SIGNS OF AGING

1. I have gained weight around my midsection (belly fat).   T/F

2. I have been told that I have bone loss/osteoporosis.   T/F

3. I have been told that I have diabetes and/or insulin resistance.   T/F

4. I'm not as strong as I used to be.   T/F

5. I'm not as muscular as I used to be.   T/F

6. I have gained 10 pounds or more over the past year.   T/F

7. I have been told that I have a high LDL cholesterol score.   T/F

8. My skin is beginning to sag. T/F

9. I have noticed reduced flexibility or increased stiffness in my joints. T/F

10. I have trouble concentrating, slow recall, and/or foggy thinking. T/F

SYMPTOMS OF AGING

1. I often feel blue or depressed. T/F

2. I feel lethargic midmorning or midafternoon. T/F

3. I often experience an overall feeling of fatigue. T/F

4. I wake up frequently during the night and experience poor sleep. T/F

5. I am not accomplishing as much as I used to at work. T/F

6. I have difficulty with sexual arousal, low libido, less intense orgasm,
   or poor erections. T/F

7. I am prone to irritability/emotional swings/anxiety. T/F

8. I lack stamina. T/F

9. I have slow recovery time after exercise. T/F

10. I train as hard as I used to, but don't get the same results. T/F

Step Two: Focus on a Heart-Centered, Healthy Aging Plan

Cardiovascular disease is the leading cause of death in the United States, and more than one in three American men currently have cardiovascular disease. Every 25 seconds an American will have a heart attack; every 40 seconds someone has a stroke; and every minute one of these men will die. The average age for a man to experience his first heart attack is 64.

Atherosclerosis is the cause of blood vessel disease that leads to heart attacks and strokes. It refers to the plaque that grows in the walls of blood vessels. Inflammation is intrinsically connected to all phases of cardiovascular disease. In fact, atherosclerosis can begin in childhood and later lead to a damaged endothelium (the thin, one-cell layer lining the interior of your vascular tree) ultimately creating plaque buildup.

Plaque is not a normal result of aging, and if you have any plaque, you have disease that needs to be aggressively treated. More than 90 percent of heart attack events occur in men with significantly diseased blood vessels at arterial sites undetectable with conventional diagnostics, such as stress testing. Stress tests pick up vascular disease that blocks the lumen of the arteries that feed your heart. It takes at least a 70 percent blockage in one of your coronary arteries to fail a stress test. Eighty-six percent of heart attacks occur with less than a 70 percent blockage. Tim Russert, the former *Meet the Press* host and NBC Washington bureau chief, is a prime example. He passed his stress test and died two months later of a heart attack caused by cholesterol plaque in the wall of one of his coronary arteries that ruptured into the lumen. He was 58 years old. This happens often because as much as 99 percent of all plaque in the artery is in the wall of the blood vessel and does not block the flow of blood.

Yet most physicians base their therapies for heart attack and stroke prevention on traditional risk-factor identification: monitoring blood pressure, cholesterol, smoking, and diabetes. But improving or eliminating risk factors alone fails to identify many men who have hidden disease. These "surprise" heart attacks and strokes can also be prevented with optimized healthcare, which is a paradigm shift away from the current status quo or standard of care, which frequently misses critical markers that could save your life. But to achieve this optimized care, you and your physician must take the right steps. The bottom line is that you need to identify blood vessel disease as early as possible in order to get the right treatment that will stop its progression.

In order to do this, make sure that your physician looks for early vascular disease and, if discovered, closely monitors your treatment with a comprehensive program that is tailored specifically for you. I have listed in Chapter 14 the testing that I believe is necessary to diagnose subclinical atherosclerosis and avoid a heart attack or stroke. For example, Carotid Intima-Media Thickness testing (CIMT) is now considered one of the best, least expensive tests to detect subclinical atherosclerosis, which allows your physician to take the right steps to halt its progression or even reverse it.

Most heart attacks and strokes occur when a blood clot forms in an inflamed artery, cutting off the blood supply to the affected heart or brain tissue. Blood clots occur when soft plaque in the wall of the artery ruptures or erodes through the lining (endothelium) of the blood vessel. There are several reliable tests for vascular inflammation that causes plaque rupture or erosion. These nontraditional blood tests are beneficial for determining whether you have blood vessel disease and how far it has progressed. They can predict your risk of a heart attack or stroke and can also be used as markers of treatment success.

Another important cause of heart attacks and strokes that many men overlook is periodontal disease, a chronic infection of the gums. At least 75 percent of men have periodontal disease. Periodontal disease can increase the risk of coronary artery disease in men less than 50 years old by 72 percent. If you have severe periodontal disease you are 3.8 times more likely to have a heart attack and twice as likely to have a stroke. Your dentist can play a major role in keeping you from having a heart attack and stroke: Be sure to see him/her often.

I believe, and the medical literature supports me, that the better care your heart gets—including the right exercise, nutrition, nutraceuticals, and healthy hormone levels—the easier it is to reduce your risk of heart disease and prevent other age-related illnesses, including diabetes, Alzheimer's, cancer, erectile dysfunction, arthritis, and other inflammatory diseases. The reactionary, traditional approach to healthcare today avoids preventive measures and moves us near the archway of death, then uses highly invasive, highly expensive treatments to pull us back, making us feel "grateful" while heart centers and hospitals reap the fiscal profits.

There are plenty of established, proactive medical protocols that are inexpensive and shown to prevent cardiovascular disease. And yet, are they promoted by cardiologists, the AMA, or health centers? Not sufficiently. As a result, many of us will undergo costly procedures, be prescribed expensive heart medication, and live less-than-desired quality lives. And quite possibly, many of us will go to emergency rooms with chest pain or die suddenly before we get to the hospital.

My proactive approach makes much more sense, since it keeps you disease free for as long as possible. It begins with positive measures, running diagnostics that uncover disease biomarkers so you can take action. And that clearly puts you in a better position to make lifestyle changes, which promote better health and diminish disease risks. Every aspect—nutrition/supplements, exercise, endocrine balance, and mind-body—must work in concert.

Since heart disease is the leading cause of death for men—and is intricately linked to erectile dysfunction—every strategy in this book is designed to help you prevent or reverse cardiovascular disorders and maintain a great sex life. I believe it's my duty as a physician to present a heart-healthy approach that proactively protects your endothelium. The endothelium forms a dynamic interface between your blood and your body. Endothelial cells secrete substances—like the important messenger molecule, nitric oxide, needed for a number of critical physiological processes—to regulate vital chemical reactions, keep blood moving smoothly, control blood pressure, ensure vascular tone, control inflammatory processes, and prevent oxidation and coagulation.

When not properly cared for, your endothelial cells become dysfunctional and fall prey to numerous disease processes, which cause atherosclerosis, hypertension, inflammatory syndromes, heart attacks, stroke, and dementia. A 2003 Mayo Clinic paper defined endothelial dysfunction as the "ultimate risk" among all the cardiovascular risk factors. If you have any of the conditions/histories listed below, you must start working very hard at improving the health of your endothelium:

- Family history of heart disease and/or confirmed heart disease, based on carotid ultrasound diagnostics, abnormal stress test, or an elevated calcium score

- History of elevated LDL levels or low HDL levels

- Elevated total cholesterol levels

- Have been diagnosed with Metabolic Syndrome (see page 32)

- Elevated triglyceride levels

- Elevated cardio CRP (C Reactive Protein) levels

- Vascular disease

Take my experience, for example. Thanks to a truly forward-thinking physician, I began undergoing periodic, proactive evaluations and, later, a carotid ultrasound, years before I should have had a heart attack. The normal protocol would have been to wait until I barely survived an emergency room visit. Instead, because of an abnormal carotid ultrasound, I was encouraged to have a 64-slice CT scan and subsequent cardiac catheterization. I learned I had chronic, yet stable heart disease involving my coronary arteries, which probably began back in my 20s. According to my cardiologist, what saved me from advanced disease and an early death was the age management medicine program I had been following for the past seven years: low-glycemic nutrition, supplements, a vital exercise regimen, and correcting my hormone deficiencies.

Further research made me realize that although the low-glycemic nutrition I had been following for years may have been good, it wasn't enough to fight or reverse heart disease. I immediately changed my whole nutritional approach to a near-vegan-style diet—blending low-glycemic foods with a strong focus on low fat. This more extreme diet approach is probably not necessary if you don't have heart disease. But if you do, then give serious thought to starting—and staying—on the Heart Health Diet outlined in Chapter 3.

Step Three: Avoid Muscle Loss

The current thinking in the medical literature is that people lose muscle mass and strength as they age—a disease called sarcopenia—and this is unavoidable. That's right, the experts believe there is nothing you or I can do to avoid losing muscle tissue and strength as we get older. I say this way of thinking is nonsense. Hasn't anyone out there ever exercised before?

The Life Plan is based on avoiding the loss of muscle tissue and strength as we age. Sarcopenia is a deadly consequence of getting old. It inflicts enormous declines in quality of life and disability on our aging population.

Sarcopenia begins in your 30s. The muscle atrophy and loss—not to mention the devastating aftermath—affect every facet of your life. If you don't exercise properly, eat right, and correct hormonal deficiencies, loss of muscle will progress at the rate of 3 percent to 5 percent with each decade starting in your 30s and 40s, then increase to 10 percent to 20 percent every decade after that. The average American male can expect to gain approximately one pound of body fat every year between ages 30 to 60 and lose about a half pound of muscle mass each year over the same time frame. At age 60 and onward it gets even worse as the rise in body fat replaces muscle mass. The largest loss of muscle mass occurs between ages 50 and 75, averaging 25 percent to 30 percent.

Aging, degenerating, and dying mitochondria are now thought to play the key role in causing sarcopenia. Mitochondria are microscopic organelles that are found inside our cells, especially muscle cells. They are the principal sites where all of our energy, in the form of ATP (adenosine triphosphate), is generated. You can thank your mom for your mitochondria, because you get them all from her. As your mitochondria age they lose their ability to produce ATP and muscle cells shrivel and die. If dying and degenerating mitochondria could be replaced with new young vibrant mitochondria, muscle and strength loss could be avoided as people age. This is exactly what the Life Plan is all about, especially my focus on exercise and resistance training.

My Life Plan focuses on the perfect combination of nutrition, the right kind of exercise, and healthy hormone levels to help you replace your old dying mitochondria with new *wild-type mitochondria*—the term scientists use (very appropriate, I might add) for young, healthy mitochondria, no matter what your age is today. This is the "fountain of youth, " in my opinion, and you'll learn more about it later in this book.

Unfortunately, most doctors devote little, if any, time to teaching patients about preventing disease. That's because most doctors do not know how to incorporate preventive medicine into their own lifestyle, let alone into their medical practice. Despite all the research pointing to the impact lifestyle has on disease prevention, medical schools continue to churn out doctors who know little if anything about how to prevent disease and preserve vitality through appropriate exercise, proper nutrition, and balanced metabolic/endocrine functions.

This is particularly evident when it comes to men's health. An October 2008 paper on low testosterone and its association with type 2 diabetes reported that androgen deficiency is a clinically underdiagnosed endocrine disorder affecting a "significant number of men in the United States and can affect up to 50 percent of men diagnosed with type 2 diabetes." Investigators in a 2004 study estimated that low testosterone deficiency affects 13.8 million men. Yet fewer than 10 percent of these men were receiving treatment.

THE LIFE PLAN'S THREE SECRETS FOR HEALTHY AGING

1. Do some form of exercise every day.

2. Make sure that everything you put in your mouth helps you instead of hurts you.

3. Make sure you do not have hormone deficiencies.

An August 2008 study demonstrated that Metabolic Syndrome, which includes obesity (especially abdominal obesity), diabetes, high blood pressure, and cholesterol problems, have a common denominator: testosterone deficiency.

Correcting testosterone deficiencies along with other hormone deficiencies in men can reverse Metabolic Syndrome and greatly improve health in many ways, from improving bone mineral density, sexual function, libido, and body fat composition to reducing risk for heart disease, diabetes, cancer, stroke, and Alzheimer's disease. An optimal level of testosterone can actually decrease or eliminate erectile dysfunction.

This is particularly important because erectile dysfunction (ED) is a window into your total health. Erectile dysfunction can be an early warning sign of underlying vascular disease and diabetes. Research reveals that many men experience erectile dysfunction four to five years before having a heart attack. Research published in 2009 from the Mayo Clinic shows that men with ED had an 80 percent higher risk for coronary artery disease. You'll learn more about all of this in Chapter 10. So if you are considering hormone therapies to improve your sex life, know that you are taking care of every aspect of your health at the same time.

However, let me make one thing crystal clear: hormone therapy is *not* the reason that I look as good as I do. In fact, it is just one integral part of my program. While they certainly help me maintain my muscle mass, it's really the combination of my diet and exercise program along with this therapy that keeps me looking fit. Together, these three aspects of the Life Plan allow me to feel younger, healthier, and sexy. There is no shortcut to optimal health, so don't make the mistake of thinking that hormone therapies are the "secret" to big muscles or a better physique.

The Time Is Now

Whether you are 26 or 76 or anywhere in between, it's not too late to get with the program. Let's get started on the Life Plan right now, by reevaluating your diet and seeing if there's room for improvement. You've got nothing to lose except the extra pounds that are slowing you down and ruining your quality of life.

CHAPTER 2

The Life Plan for Healthy Eating

- -

A s a physician, I'm fully aware that the foods we choose to eat profoundly affect our physical and mental health, our athletic performance, and how we age. Researchers are continuing to uncover the direct links between food choices and the frightening increase in diseases such as diabetes, heart disease, and obesity. Yet as a man, just knowing that certain foods will make me sick, and certainly make me look and feel older, is often not enough to stop me from eating things I know are bad for me.

Nutrition has always been the toughest aspect of my own personal health journey. I accomplished my health goals in spite of my bad habits and my tendency to make bad decisions about what I put into my mouth. Before my transformation, I ate too many of the wrong foods all the time, and way too much of them—breads, white rice, French fries, ice cream, any and all chocolates, all kinds of sweets, lots of red meat, fried foods; the list goes on and on. Like most men, I'm still battling with a borderline consumption disorder, and it doesn't end with food. I'm the first to admit that I can easily drink way too much. The potbelly and added pounds I was carrying thirteen years ago were directly linked to eating too much poor-quality protein, starch, fats, and sugar, and drinking too much alcohol.

Even to this day, if I start eating the wrong foods it isn't long before I'm completely off track. I know that in order to keep myself trim and feeling young, I need to completely cut out all the wrong foods from my diet and get them out of my house. I know that having my pantry, refrigerator, and freezer loaded up with unhealthy foods, even if they are supposed to be for someone else in my family, creates a toxic food environment for me.

My experience with eating is similar to that of most of my patients. The most vulnerable area in every man's effort to change his body and his life seems to always be diet. It's the deal breaker for just about everybody. But I know that if you can win the eating battle, you can win the war against excess body fat and poor health.

The first step to winning this war is to understand why you need to lose weight in the first place. Then, you'll learn how to choose the best foods to improve your health and achieve your fat-loss goals. The goal for my Life Plan is to get you in the best shape possible, starting with your diet. If you avoid the foods that can make you sick as well as fat you'll see a complete reversal in the signs and symptoms of aging, and you will drop those unnecessary, unhealthy pounds and increase your metabolism and energy levels.

THE LIFE PLAN NUTRITION GOALS

- Prevent disease

- Increase metabolism and energy

- Control appetite

- Enhance natural hormone levels

Prevent Disease

Whether you are seven or 70 pounds overweight, those extra pounds of fat can spell trouble for your health and your sex life. First, maintaining a healthy weight now will reduce cognitive decline later on. A study in the March 2009 issue of *Archives of Neurology* investigated whether total and/or regional body fat levels influence cognitive decline. Researchers found that in men, worsening cognitive function correlated with the highest levels of all adiposity measures: The fatter you are, the more likely you will experience cognitive decline later in life.

What's more, your weight affects every aspect of how your body functions. Obesity is such an enormous epidemic that we've created a new name for an old problem: Metabolic Syndrome, also known as Syndrome X. As many as 75 million Americans are now believed to be affected. Simply put, Metabolic Syndrome occurs when excess weight affects your health, particularly your heart, as well as your body's ability to process sugar, leading to diabetes. The four key components of Metabolic Syndrome are obesity (especially abdominal obesity), diabetes or insulin resistance, elevated triglyceride levels (one of the fats in the blood), high blood pressure, and increased silent inflammation. There can also be other abnormalities as part of this syndrome, including elevated total cholesterol levels, elevated LDL (the bad cholesterol) levels, low levels of HDL (the good cholesterol), and elevated levels of fibrinogen (a protein that promotes dangerous blood clot formation). Each of these components can also be linked to sexual dysfunction.

Now for the good news—Metabolic Syndrome is completely and totally preventable and reversible. Weight loss, exercise, and correcting hormone deficiencies are the keys to preventing this disease. And, if you already have the syndrome, exercise will also correct the abnormalities that characterize the disease by improving insulin receptor sensitivity. The key is to lose body fat—especially abdominal fat.

It turns out that when body fat is stored mostly in your abdomen, health risks skyrocket. Abdominal obesity is a common problem for almost all men. It results mostly from fat being deposited inside the abdominal cavity—the so-called intra-abdominal fat or visceral fat. Unfortunately, this is the worst kind of fat to have because it not only adds inches to your waistline, it's one of the major causes of Metabolic Syndrome.

This kind of fat doesn't just hang out quietly, like the fat on your arms and legs or under your skin (subcutaneous fat). Abdominal fat is very much alive, actively producing harmful proinflammatory molecules called adipokines and other chemicals that cause atherosclerosis, cancer, elevated blood sugars, and insulin resistance, and contribute to silent inflammation that can occur in many places throughout the body. The reasons for this aren't fully understood, but many experts think that intra-abdominal fat produces not only harmful hormones but also free fatty acids much more easily than subcutaneous fat. These free fatty acids are directly transported to your liver, where they can interfere with insulin metabolism and create a state of hyperinsulinemia (high insulin levels), poor blood sugar control, salt retention, high blood pressure, and silent inflammation—all major causes of disease and hormone deficiencies.

Silent Inflammation

Silent inflammation is the most insidious form of inflammation because it is the root of almost all diseases. You can't feel it. It's an insidious killer many experts consider to be the major culprit in accelerating the aging process and causing age-related disease. Dr. Barry Sears, a leader in this field of medicine, was one of the first to point out the important role diet plays in both causing and preventing silent inflammation. I have incorporated many of his recommendations into my Life Nutrition Plan.

Insulin Resistance

Insulin resistance is the central problem of Metabolic Syndrome and is associated with chronically elevated levels of insulin and blood sugars (although blood sugars can be normal, especially early in the disease). Many researchers believe that high levels of insulin cause the other components of Metabolic Syndrome to develop—obesity, high triglycerides, elevated blood pressure, and inflammation. Excess levels of insulin are also thought to be the single most important factor in accelerating the aging process. High insulin levels affect your body fat percentage, blood lipid levels, glucose tolerance, aerobic capacity, muscle mass, strength, and immune function. What's more, insulin resistance is present in most people with cardiovascular disease.

Insulin not only regulates blood sugar, it also plays a very important role in fat metabolism by increasing the secretion of lipoprotein lipase, which increases the uptake of fat from your bloodstream into body cells. So, when insulin levels are kept low you reduce your risk for all of the serious diseases most Americans die from, and you are much less likely to convert calories into body fat.

The major cause of insulin resistance is poor nutrition and lack of exercise. As your body fat increases, your insulin receptor sensitivity plummets. As insulin sensitivity drops, insulin secretion from your pancreas increases, triggering a multitude of changes, which include damage to the lining of your heart's blood vessels (endothelial dysfunction), interference with the enzymes that break down fats in your blood, and interference with your kidney's ability to get rid of sodium (causing high blood pressure).

Remember, the more resistant you are to your insulin, the more insulin your body needs to make in order to maintain your blood sugar levels. And more insulin equals more body fat. Both aerobic and resistance training have been shown to reverse insulin resistance. The more you burn fat for energy (as opposed to glycogen) during your aerobic training the more sensitive you become to the insulin your body produces. As your body fat disappears and your muscle mass increases, your insulin resistance diminishes, taking a huge burden off your pancreas, so that it can now secrete less insulin throughout the day. The greater your sensitivity is to insulin, the more effective you become at removing sugar from your blood and tapping into your fat stores for your energy needs. You also reduce your need and desire for consuming extra calories because your body can now tap into stored body fat more efficiently. It's physiologically impossible for you to burn your body fat for energy when your insulin levels are high.

Controlling insulin levels is the primary objective of my nutrition plan. This can best be achieved by eating small meals and carefully controlling your intake of carbohydrates, limiting your choices to those with a low glycemic index (most vegetables and fruits, and a few of the whole grains). It is also important to always eat a high-quality, low-fat source of protein with any carbohydrate we consume. The ratio (gram/gram) of protein to carbohydrate needed to achieve ideal insulin control is between 0.5 and 1.0. Diets that stay in this range are proven to result in a greater loss of body fat than diets with ratios below 0.5. Nutritional programs with protein-to-carbohydrate ratios below 0.5 are the high-carbohydrate diets promoted by the USDA Food Pyramid, the American Heart Association, and Dr. Dean Ornish. They all result in excess insulin production and elevated fasting insulin levels—the root cause of heart disease and the obesity epidemic.

A recent study in the *American Journal of Nutrition* compared diets with the same number of calories but different protein-to-carb ratios. The diet with a protein-to-carbohydrate ratio of 0.6 (similar to my Life Nutrition Plan) keeps insulin levels low and maintains a positive nitrogen balance. The diet higher in carbohydrates and lower in protein, such as the American Heart Association Diet (with a protein-to-carbohydrate ratio of 0.25), tends to increase insulin secretion and produce a negative nitrogen balance. A negative nitrogen balance means you are breaking down your muscles to provide energy for your body. A positive nitrogen balance, on the other hand, indicates that you are building muscle mass.

As caloric requirements are reduced, you will find that you are eating less food and thereby reducing the number of free radicals (the unstable atoms that are produced when food is converted to energy) produced when these foods are digested and stored. Many scientists believe that if we can reduce free-radical production in our bodies, we will reduce the damage they do to our cells and dramatically slow the aging process. In addition to exercise, watching your overall calorie intake is the only proven way to slow the aging process to date.

Lastly, when you structure your nutrition program around keeping blood sugars and insulin levels in check, you will get another big benefit—increased muscle size. In just four to seven days of eating "clean, " you will have your blood sugar and insulin levels in the ideal metabolic range, and by two weeks you will no longer be plagued by feelings of hunger, deprivation, and cravings. You'll experience a marked improvement in your mental focus, exercise endurance, strength, optimal health, muscularity, and leanness.

Glycation

Another problem with elevated blood sugars is glycation (or glycosylation), the process in which sugar molecules floating around our bloodstream become attached to proteins and nucleic acids and produce new, and very dangerous, chemical structures. Ninety-nine percent of all cellular activities depend on a vast array of proteins in our bodies, and when sugars bind to them they become dysfunctional and create major problems.

These glycated proteins are called advanced glycation end-products (AGEs), and they attack collagen (used to make ligaments, tendons, and other connective tissue vital for muscle strength and growth) and nucleic acids, which are vital to the synthesis of new proteins. Glycated proteins become very "sticky" and adhere to the inside walls of blood vessels, causing endothelial dysfunction, which leads to vascular dysfunction—the inability of the artery to properly dilate and constrict. This causes the buildup of plaque, which obstructs blood flow to our hearts, brains, hands, feet, eyes, muscles, the penis, and other vital organs. Over time the function of all of our cells and arteries becomes seriously compromised, with significant health consequences, including both mental and physical deterioration.

Glycation is an entirely passive process and does not require any chemical reaction. It is simply dependent on the number of sugar molecules in our bloodstream—the more there are, the more AGEs we form and the more we pollute our bodies.

Glycation is considered one of the most significant biological markers of aging. Many authorities believe that glycation is most responsible for the development of degenerative disease. Glycation is also associated with chronically elevated insulin levels. Insulin not only promotes central obesity (big bellies) but also prevents our fat cells from converting their stored fat into the free fatty acids that we can use for our energy needs. Because we are unable to tap into this huge energy reservoir, we get tired and hungry between meals when our blood sugars are low, and we are subsequently driven to eat more sugar-containing foods to satisfy our energy needs.

This promotes a vicious cycle of unstable blood sugars, elevated insulin levels, high rates of glycation, and uncontrolled eating, which persists and actually worsens over time. Slowly we poison our metabolic systems and hurt each and every one of our cells and our arteries.

The amount of glycation that is occurring in your body can be measured by the Hemoglobin A1C test mentioned in Chapter 1. You want your value to be between 4.0 and 5.5 percent—the lower the better. Typical levels seen in type 2 diabetics are between 8 and 11 percent. If your level is between 5.7 and 6.4 you are likely to be insulin resistant. Glycation levels are directly related to the speed at which you are aging—the higher they are, the faster you are going to age and the greater risk you have for developing an age-related disease.

When glycation rates are controlled and kept low by the right nutrition and exercise programs, insulin levels are also kept low. In the face of low insulin levels we can tap into the huge energy storage depot in our bodies (our own body fat) for our energy needs, and before we know it, we become lean, muscular, and healthy. This is truly a winning situation not only because we look and feel great, but because excess body fat is another very important biological marker of aging and disease.

If you follow my specific nutritional recommendations in combination with my exercise program you can minimize glycation and add 10 to 15 years to your life. That is, 10 to 15 more years of vitality, productivity, and great health—not 10 to 15 more years in a nursing home.

Calculating Your Weight Loss Goals

The first and easiest measurement you need to know is the actual size of your spare tire. This alone has been shown to be a better predictor of future heart attacks and type 2 diabetes than body mass index. It is very easy to determine if you have too much intra-abdominal fat, and you don't need any fancy, high-priced laboratory tests to do it. All you need is an inexpensive cloth tape measure. Simply measure your abdominal girth, or waist circumference. And I don't mean the "low waist, " where most of us wear our pants, but rather the "high waist"—at your belly button, where you are the largest. If your waist circumference is forty inches or greater your risk for life-threatening disease increases dramatically. Remember that visceral fat is the first place you gain . . . and the last place you drop the weight. But don't get discouraged—you can get rid of stubborn belly fat, just as I have, by following the Life Plan.

Next, you need to know your current weight. Simple enough: Step on a scale. But this number isn't enough. Most healthcare professionals rely on a formula called the body mass index

(BMI), which takes into account your current weight and height to determine whether you are overweight. This index is calculated by multiplying your weight in pounds by 705, dividing the result by your height in inches, and then dividing again by your height in inches. If your BMI is between 25 and 30 you are considered heavy, and if it is greater than 30 you're obese. Currently, BMI is also used by doctors, nutritionists, and other health professionals to assess health risks.

This simplified approach works fairly well when we look at large populations, but because it takes into account only weight and height, it misses what really is increasing your risk for diabetes, strokes, cancer, arthritis, and premature death—"fatness."

Being overweight is not the problem. Being overfat is. Overfat means carrying around too much body fat, which is actually what profoundly influences our health, physical and mental performance, and appearance. Every man who is muscular is considered overweight according to the BMI, even if he is lean—because of his increased muscle weight. At the same time, there are plenty of men who have a great BMI but have way too much fat and very little muscle mass. Unfortunately, almost 70 percent of adults in the United States are considered fat. It is the second leading cause of preventable death in the United States, and will soon be the first; smoking is still more deadly than fatness.

Many doctors agree with me that the measurement we should be focusing on is our percentage of body fat. This can help us determine an individual's ideal body weight, degree of fatness, and risk for disease. In the following table, I have listed the percentages of body fat for men according to their age that correlate with excellent to poor health/fitness ratings. This can be used as a general guideline to help you achieve your ideal body weight.

PERCENTAGE OF BODY FAT FOR MEN

Health/Fitness Rating	Ages 20–29	Ages 30–39	Ages 40–49	Ages 50–59	Ages 60+
Excellent	<11	<12	<14	<15	<16
Good	11–13	12–14	14–16	15–17	16–18
Average	14–20	15–21	17–23	18–24	19–25
Fair	21–23	22–24	24–26	25–27	26–28
Poor	>23	>24	>26	>27	>28

You can measure your body fat in any number of ways, but the most common tool is skin-fold calipers. You can buy your own or get tested at your local gym. However, the results are only as good as the tester. The test requires someone else to determine the thickness of skin folds at various sites on your body. The measurements are then plugged into an equation to determine your body fat percentage. But there are more than 100 different calculations to choose from. Make sure that your tester is using the most accurate equation, or you may come up with a result that is completely misleading.

The gold standard for measuring body fat percentage is the DEXA scan, which many doctors like me can perform right in their office. A DEXA scan also tells how many grams of muscle tissue you have, so it can track gains in muscle mass resulting from your fat-loss/muscle-building program.

ONE PHOTO IS ALL IT TAKES

My best motivator during my transformation was my "before" photo that I sent to the Body-*for*-LIFE competition. Every time I didn't feel like dieting or exercising, I would just look at that photo of myself on my boat and remember how much I didn't want to be that man anymore. So take a photo of yourself today, keep it in your cell phone or in your wallet, and look at it often. For the most honest assessment, take the picture wearing a Speedo: It's probably the only time you will ever wear one.

Body fat of more than 25 percent puts men in the obese, high-health-risk category. As a general rule, I believe that no man at any age should have greater than 15 percent body fat if he wants to remain optimally fit and healthy. At age 72, I work very hard at keeping my body fat below 10 percent, and at this percentage, I feel the best, have far greater energy, move better, think better, look my best, and have the lowest risk for disease.

Track What You Eat

Your genetics do set the lower limits for your desirable and achievable weight, but the decisions you make regarding your food and exercise are what will ultimately affect your weight loss. The first step in losing body fat is keeping an accurate account of what you eat every day. For one week, record in the food journal I've provided in Chapter 8 every little bite and gulp and calculate the number of calories you consume every day, by working off the calorie information on food packages. The caloric value of fresh foods, such as fruits and vegetables, and proteins are readily available on several diet and nutrition websites like mine, www.DrLife.com. At the end of one week, total up the calories you have eaten and divide by 7 to get your average daily caloric intake. This number gives you the precise number of calories you need on a daily basis to maintain your present weight.

Since your goal is to lose weight, you need to decrease this number by 20 percent. Multiply your current daily average by 20 percent, and then subtract this result from your present daily average to get your new daily calorie limit.

It's important that you not decrease your intake by more than 20 percent, because this will put you into a muscle-losing, slow-metabolism mode. If you are one of those fortunate few men who need to gain weight, just reverse by adding 10 to 20 percent to your average daily caloric intake. You will start packing on the weight before you know it, and if you do so while following the exercise program, you'll gain muscle instead of body fat.

Next, you need to calculate the number of calories you need from fat. Take your new daily calorie count and multiply it by 15 percent: This will give you the number of fat calories your body requires. Divide this number by 9 to convert fat calories into grams of fat.

Then, you need to calculate the number of calories of protein you will need to maximize your muscle-building efforts. Simply take 1 gram per pound of your body weight and multiply this number by 4 (4 calories per gram of protein), and this will give you the number of protein calories you need each day.

Add your protein calories to your fat calories and subtract this amount from your new total daily caloric limit to get the number of calories of carbohydrates you should eat. Carbohydrate calories can be converted to grams by dividing by 4 (4 calories per gram of carbohydrate).

For example, my patient Tony was a 190-pound, 45-year-old male. Here's how I came up with his caloric needs:

Present daily caloric intake	2, 800 cal
20%	560 cal
New daily caloric limit	2, 240 cal

FAT REQUIREMENTS

15% fat calories	336 cal
Fat calories/9 = gm of fat	37 gm

PROTEIN REQUIREMENTS

1 gm/pound of body weight	190 gm
190 gm x 4 cal/gm	760 cal

COMPOSITION OF NEW DAILY NUTRITION PLAN

Protein 190 gm	760 cal
Fat 37 gm	336 cal
Carbs 378 gm	1,144 cal
Total	2,240 cal

Are You Resistant to Fat Loss?

Occasionally some men reach a plateau in their fat-loss program, and they just can't drop any more body fat. It is rare for my patients to not lose weight on my program, but it's fairly common for men to reach a sticking point just short of their ultimate fat-loss goal. They just can't seem to get past it even in the face of extreme caloric restriction.

This resistance to fat loss can be caused by several factors, including medications. Psychotropic drugs are the major culprits, and they include antidepressants and antianxiety agents. Hormone or hormonelike medications, including prednisone, are also contributors to this metabolic resistance syndrome. Cardiovascular, blood pressure, diuretic, and antiarthritic (NSAIDs) drugs can also produce metabolic resistance. If you are taking a medication that you think may be contributing to your failure to lose body fat, don't just stop taking it. Talk it over with your doctor and see if an alternative can be used that won't adversely affect your fat-loss efforts.

If medications aren't the problem, make sure you don't have an underactive thyroid gland. The tests listed in Chapter 14 can help you determine if you need to take thyroid hormone replacement medication to correct your resistance to weight loss. And if medications and thyroid problems aren't the cause of your metabolic resistance syndrome, then modify your nutrition plan. Begin eating slightly fewer calories. If, after a week, you still haven't broken through your sticking point, then slowly begin replacing some carbohydrate calories with more healthy fats (including foods high in omega-3 and -6 fatty acids, which I'll discuss later) and protein. It's very likely that if you stay at that ratio of fat and protein to carbohydrates you will begin seeing the fat disappear right before your eyes.

Increase Metabolism and Energy

Metabolism is the energy we expend to maintain all physical and chemical changes in our body. Our metabolic rate reflects how rapidly we use our energy stores. This rate is influenced by many factors, including our genetics, natural hormonal activity, body size, and body fat composition. While we can't change our genetics, we can control all of the other factors that influence our metabolism. It's also interesting to know that contrary to popular belief, your age has a minimal effect on your metabolic rate. Instead, it's your hormone levels and level of fitness that are the key components. For example, I once calculated the basal metabolic rate (BMR) of a 20-year-old male weighing 154 pounds, and compared that to a 60-year-old male weighing the same. The 20-year-old's resting energy expenditure was 1,750 calories per day, and the 60-year-old's was 1,691 calories per day—only 59 calories less. The key to the older man's success was that he was actively maintaining his healthy hormone levels.

The second secret to keeping your metabolism running is simple: You need muscle. The more muscle or lean body mass you have, the greater the number of calories you will burn throughout the day. You can improve your muscle mass through exercise (both resistance training and aerobic exercise), which can dramatically increase your daily energy expenditure and burn off excess body fat. If the exercise is intense enough, you will continue to burn extra calories throughout the day.

Metabolism Is Influenced by Food Choices

It takes energy, in the form of calories, for the body to metabolize food. This is called diet-induced thermogenesis (DIT). DIT is the amount of energy (calories) the body uses to digest, metabolize, and store the foods we eat. We know that it takes more energy to digest and convert proteins and complex carbohydrates (up to 25 percent of the meal's total calories) than for fats and sugars. So it makes sense for us to focus on meals that are high in protein and complex carbs, which will burn off more efficiently and leave fewer calories for storage. High DIT foods include chicken, turkey, lean red meats, brown rice, wild rice, yams, vegetables, apples, and other nontropical fruits. Foods that have a low DIT include all processed foods that are high in carbohydrates and fat (like the ones found in most fast-food restaurants), white bread, white rice, French fries—in other words, most of the things we all love to eat.

High DIT meals burn more calories than meals with low DIT even when they both have the same number of calories. For example, a plain peanut butter sandwich on whole grain bread may have the same calories as a ham sandwich with mayonnaise on white bread. However, the peanut butter sandwich is better for you, because it has a higher DIT. Ideally, if we want to get leaner, each of our meals should be designed to maximize its DIT.

Better still, DIT calories are burned without our having to do anything, because we have to eat and digest our food in order to survive. By choosing the right foods, you can potentially lose weight without even trying. You can also maximize your DIT by choosing when to eat. Since DIT is greatest just one hour after eating, it makes sense to eat frequently throughout the day. That's why I suggest that you have five or six small meals a day, so that you can take advantage of the increased metabolic rate that accompanies eating.

The foods on the Life Plan are chosen specifically for their ability to increase your energy by supplying your body with the nutrients it needs. Not only will increasing your metabolism make you feel more alive and awake every day, but you will also be training your body to burn food more efficiently, creating more energy to literally pump up your workouts and eliminate body fat. This is the good kind of vicious cycle: When you increase your energy, you'll have more energy to exercise, which in turn increases your metabolism to burn more food, leaving you leaner and healthier.

There Is a Right Time to Eat

A 1993 study by Romon et al., published in the 57th edition of the *American Journal of Clinical Nutrition,* researched the relationship between DIT and the time meals were eaten. These scientists were able to demonstrate that if a meal is eaten in the morning, 16 percent of its calories are used to metabolize the meal. When the same meal was eaten in the afternoon, 13.5 percent of its calories were needed to metabolize the food. When the meal was eaten at night, only 10.9 percent of its calories were used to metabolize the food. In other words, if you eat a meal at night rather than in the morning or afternoon, you lose the benefit of the thermogenic response you would have gotten earlier in the day. You are allowing foods with high DIT calories to be stored as body fat rather than being used by your body to process the food. This is clearly a problem in America, since most men consume the largest proportion of their calories in the evening.

On the Life Plan, you will consume the majority of your calories by 6:00 or 7:00 P.M. If you must eat after that, choose lean proteins (a small piece of chicken, or a tablespoon or two of peanut butter, for example) and avoid fats and carbohydrates. Only 3 percent of fat calories are used for DIT, while 23 percent of carbohydrate calories and a whopping 30 percent of protein calories are burned as a result of DIT.

For the best muscle-building and fat-burning potential, you will need to eat within one hour after your workout. The exercise has done its job of stimulating your muscle growth. Now protein and carbohydrates are needed in the right combination to promote the ideal hormonal conditions for maximum growth. It is these nutrients that trigger the release of insulin and growth hormone, which move valuable amino acids and carbs into your muscle cells.

The best food to consume immediately after a strength-training workout is 12 ounces of a liquid protein/carbohydrate drink. The drink should consist of 0.7 grams of a high-glycemic-index carb per pound of body weight (about 100 to 140 grams) and 0.2 grams of protein per pound of body weight (about 30 to 40 grams). Carbohydrates should be high-nutritious, high-glycemic-index sources such as fruits (bananas, strawberries, oranges, and so on) and honey. This is the only time I recommend eating a high-glycemic food (more about the glycemic index later). Protein sources can include nonfat milk, nonfat yogurt, soy milk, and protein powder supplements.

ONLINE GROCERY SHOPPING

A great way I have found to make sure I have the right food at home and in my office is to avoid shopping at grocery stores and shop online instead. A 2007 study in the *International Journal of Behavioral Nutrition and Physical Activity* found that buying groceries online not only reduces unhealthy choices from impulse buying, but also helps you budget better.

Control Your Appetite

We have been programmed to believe that food is good and more is even better. Our thoughts and feelings about food have been implanted in our brains by our parents, our culture, and Madison Avenue advertising executives. In addition, the genetic code we have inherited from our ancestors that enabled them to survive in the face of severe deprivation compels us to eat high-calorie and low-volume foods even when we are not hungry, preparing us for a future famine that never comes. That's why just about every guy is plagued with occasional or even frequent episodes of a complete loss of control in terms of food.

This has created a culture of men who have consumption disorders, also known as food addiction. Literally hundreds of thousands of men have become addicted to food. You may be one of them. Take the following test and see where you stand. If your answer to many of these questions is "yes" then consider yourself one of an ever-increasing number of us (yes, I used to be) who have become carbohydrate addicts. I am proud to say that I am now a recovering food addict.

Are You a Food Addict?

According to G. Douglas Talbott, M.D., a noted authority on addiction, food addiction involves "the compulsive pursuit of a mood change by engaging repeatedly in episodes of binge eating despite adverse consequences." Food addiction is not a result of a weak will or a behavioral problem. Rather, it's a metabolic or biochemical disorder that produces all of the characteristic signs and symptoms of addiction. The irony is that food addicts eat foods to feel better that actually make them feel worse.

If you are a food addict, don't be discouraged. The first step in conquering this addiction is to recognize that you have the problem. You can then begin taking the necessary steps to get your eating under control—the absolute key to permanent fat loss and great health.

Take this simple quiz. If you answer "yes" to more than eight of these questions, you may have a diagnosable food addiction.

1. Have you ever thought that food is a problem for you?

2. Have you ever tried to cut down or control your use of sweet foods?

3. Do you eat more sweet foods than you used to?

4. Have you noticed an increased sensitivity to sweet or white flour foods resulting in increased irritability, tiredness, and depression?

5. Are you preoccupied with certain foods and the thoughts of food?

6. Do you hide wrappers?

7. Has your eating ever interfered with any part of your life?

8. Do you keep your feelings about food and eating a secret?

9. Has your weight gone up and down over the years?

10. Have you ever lied about how much sweet food or other carbs you eat?

11. Have you ever binged on sweets or white flour foods?

12. Is it impossible to "just say no" to sweet foods and other processed carbohydrates?

13. Do you frequently eat more than you planned to eat?

14. Have you hidden food so that you could have it later?

15. Have you felt angry when someone ate your special food you saved for yourself?

16. Do you worry sometimes that you cannot control how much you eat?

17. Do you gobble down certain foods rapidly, with little chewing?

18. Do you fast in order to avoid eating foods you cannot control?

19. Do you overdo exercise to make up for overeating?

20. Have you ever gone way out of your way to get something sweet?

Avoid Trigger Foods

We can beat food addictions by using a powerful tool: avoidance. Just as people with food allergies know that they can't eat certain foods or they will have a reaction, you may have the same relationship with certain foods, only this time the reaction is that they cause you to eat more. Potato chips, French fries, bagels, ice cream, cookies, bread, and fast food are all "trigger" foods. Trigger foods are the ones that you can't "have just one" of. People prefer and crave different trigger foods because of our individualized brain chemistry and even genetic makeup. Typically, trigger foods contain high levels of sugar, fat, or flour. It's quite rare for brussels sprouts, chicken breasts, broccoli, and asparagus to fall into the trigger food category.

Trigger foods stimulate the same circuits in our brains that are activated by pleasure-producing mind-altering drugs, or other addictive behavior, such as sex. In fact, many researchers believe trigger foods are truly addictive for many people because they invoke a loss of control that duplicates the behavioral consequences of addiction.

The only way to maintain control over trigger foods is by totally eliminating them from your nutrition plan. Don't deceive yourself: You will never be able to control a trigger food. The idea that you can just have "a little" never works! This is why 75 percent of dieters who are able to lose fat gain it all back in 12 to 18 months. When people reach their goal weight, most of them think they have gained control over their trigger foods. But trigger foods always win. You can never control them unless you learn to retrain your brain (see Chapter 9 for more on that).

The return to full-blown addiction is slow and very insidious, but, before you know it, you will be back to eating as much or more of your trigger food than ever before. Because of this, on the Life Plan, there is no room for a "free day" when you can eat whatever you want. The secret to getting lean and staying lean is to gain total control over your eating—and never lose it.

Social events and holidays will inevitably come up and will test your willpower. To control your eating behavior when you are at parties, you must create an eating strategy before you get there, and then stick to it. Rehearse in your mind just how you are going to deal with the foods and beverages offered. And when you do arrive—don't get there hungry. Fifteen minutes before I leave for an event I have a rounded tablespoon of Metamucil in an 8-ounce glass of water. Metamucil is psyllium, a nonsoluble fiber, which mixes with the foods you are about to eat, thereby slowing the speed of digestion and the release of sugars into your bloodstream. This really slows the entire process of eating way down and can give you the extra edge you need for staying in control.

If your hosts insist on forcing one of their dishes on you, tell them that your doctor has you on a special nutrition plan to correct a potentially lethal medical condition (fatness—but you don't have to tell them that). Then, eat only the healthiest options and avoid at all costs your trigger foods. Stay away from hors d'oeuvres that you can't account for because you are eating one at a time, and not filling a plate. If you start obsessing over one of your trigger foods, tell a friend that you've made a commitment to get lean and healthy. This will make it less likely that you will allow yourself to get caught shoving something into your mouth.

There's No Such Thing as a "Free Day" on the Life Plan

Many popular diets allow you to take a day off from eating right. This so-called free day isn't free at all. In fact, I guarantee that you'll pay for it later. The U.S. government found when it reviewed all the different weight-loss plans that within one year, 66 percent of dieters gain back all the weight they lost, and 97 percent gain it all back within five years. These numbers point out just how vulnerable we all are to trigger foods.

In my opinion, free days need to be handled with extreme caution; better still, avoid them altogether. What you eat on your free day depends entirely on your personality, your eating history, and just how much control you have over your eating. We all have very different abilities to control eating, many of which have been influenced by culture, physiology, psychology, genes, environment, brain chemistry, and the sensitivity of our taste buds. If you are overfat because you have always had a problem with control (like most of us), and if you recognize that you're especially vulnerable to trigger foods, then you simply can't afford a free day.

I know that we aren't perfect, so I can't expect you to follow this diet perfectly every day. In all honesty, I cheat every once in a while. But at the same time, I know that if I take a free day, I'll lose control for a whole lot longer. Instead, if I mess up and eat something that I shouldn't, the very next meal I'll get right back on track. So instead of thinking about a free day, I have a "free" meal once a week at the most. And I try very hard to make sure that I completely avoid trigger foods that cause me to lose control.

I also try not to eat foods that I know are bad for my health, such as French fries and fast food in general. A recent scientific study by Rudolph, published in the *American Journal of Nutrition* in August 2007, showed that in the four-hour period following eating a high-fat meal (for example, a Sausage McMuffin® with Egg/two hash browns or a Big Mac® with fries) there is a 70 percent drop in overall blood flow (because your arteries constrict, offering less elasticity), a 125 percent hike in triglycerides, a 50 percent jump in leukocytes (inflammatory white blood cells), and a 125 percent rise in IL-8 (an inflammatory marker). These changes are all a result of the immediate impact high-saturated-fat foods have on the endothelial lining of blood vessels and the heart.

Avoid Emotional Eating

The key to losing weight, and keeping it off forever, is not to follow a diet, but rather, a healthy nutrition program for the rest of your life. You must continually monitor your eating and exercise programs daily, weekly, monthly, and yearly in order to watch for pitfalls resulting from stress, negative thinking, or lifestyle changes—all of which can easily sabotage your success.

Bob Greene writes, in his book *Get with the Program*, that if there is a secret to permanent weight loss, it is the complete elimination of emotional eating. I couldn't agree more. Emotional eating occurs when we eat because of something we are feeling instead of actually being hungry. As you might guess, the causes of emotional eating can be very complex, and the successful elimination of this destructive behavior requires making significant changes in your life. These changes can be as simple as developing creative ways to handle stress or as involved as entering a psychological counseling program.

The four most common reasons for emotional eating are:

- Boredom

- Stress

- Loneliness

- Turmoil arising from childhood trauma

Emotional eating can occur at any time—during meals, at the end of meals, between meals, at social occasions, and late at night. Eliminating emotional eating from our lives is as important as (and maybe even more important than) a well-planned exercise and nutrition program in achieving and maintaining a lean, muscular, healthy body.

The first step in eliminating emotional eating is to make eating a conscious activity. Eating must always be organized and well planned. Again, keeping a food journal can really help in achieving this goal. The next step is learning to distinguish where physical hunger ends and emotional eating begins. Once this point is identified, you can then begin the hard work of taking a clear and objective look at your life and start making the changes needed for permanently eliminating emotional eating. It takes a lot of courage to get to the root cause of emotional eating, but the result will be a permanent change in the way we use food—a change that will guarantee a lifetime of leanness, fitness, and great physical and mental health—goals definitely worth achieving.

If all of these strategies fail and you find yourself reaching for your favorite trigger food, which will most assuredly lead you back down the path to fatness, reach instead for your "before picture" for an instant reality check.

Nighttime Munchies Are a Sign of Illness

If you have trouble controlling your eating after dinner, or wake up in the middle of the night to eat, you may be suffering from night-eating syndrome (NES). This syndrome is associated with both obesity and chronic fatigue. NES may be the direct result of an overreaction to stress, since we know that the stress hormone cortisol is much higher in the evening and during the night in men who have NES than in those who do not.

Nighttime awakenings with subsequent eating are very common with individuals who have NES. The food consumed is usually high-glycemic-index carbohydrates, which researchers believe is your unconscious attempt to restore the disrupted sleep cycle by increasing serotonin levels in the brain.

The key to managing this syndrome is to develop strategies to lower cortisol levels, which you can begin by systematically eliminating or decreasing as much stress in your daily life as you can. Cognitive-behavioral methods are believed to be some of the most effective techniques available for reducing and managing stress. They include identifying the sources of stress in your life, restructuring your priorities, changing your response to stress, and finally, finding methods to manage and reduce or totally eliminate the stress.

If you are afflicted with this syndrome, find a psychologist who is well trained in cognitive-behavioral therapy. Work with him or her to develop the skills you need to manage your stress and high cortisol levels. This will not only improve your life but help you gain control over your eating.

Restore Natural Hormone Levels

One of the goals of any health program is to develop a lifestyle that will enable you to increase your own production of hormones, including human growth hormone (hGH). hGH is measured as IGF-1 (Insulin-like Growth Factor-1). As the name implies, "Insulin-like Growth Factor-1" is structurally related to insulin. These two hormones share the same receptor sites on cells, creating a competition in which only one hormone will be predominantly effective. A nutrition program that focuses on keeping insulin levels as low as possible will enable you to increase your own natural production of IGF-1.

Because you need to optimize growth hormone levels and IGF-1 levels to achieve great health, increase your sex drive, and improve your quality of life, my plan is designed to keep blood sugars low, allowing you to effectively manage your insulin, which will help you achieve healthy levels of growth hormone and IGF-1 on your own.

Rules for Following the Life Plan for Healthy Eating

I have created three basic rules to help keep you on the right nutrition track:

Rule One: Meal Frequency

Rule Two: Proper Macronutrient Ratios

Rule Three: Plan Your Day

Rule One: Meal Frequency

The only way to lose body fat is to achieve a caloric deficit, either by decreasing your intake of food or by burning more calories through exercise. Exercise is, by far, the best way to achieve a caloric deficit, because it does not trigger the starvation response, it increases metabolic rate, it increases all of the fat-burning enzymes and hormones, it targets body fat rather than muscle tissue for energy sources, and it increases the sensitivity of all cells to insulin so that carbohydrates are burned for energy and stored as glycogen rather than being stored as body fat.

Scientific studies continue to reinforce the notion that the best way to eat if you want to get rid of body fat, gain muscle, reduce your risks for heart disease and other serious degenerative diseases, and not get old is to eat five to six small, balanced meals every day. When your body is presented with too much fuel at any given meal, it will store it as body fat for later use. And if you continue to take in too many calories at each meal, your body will never learn how to access this stored fuel, and body fat will continue to accumulate in your body.

Instead of eating the traditional three square meals a day, you need to trick your body by eating several low-calorie meals (200–400 calories each) every few hours. This constant feeding technique forces your body to process foods as you eat them, and then use these calories for energy before they can build up as fat in your fat cells. This technique is hands down the single most important nutritional concept for ultimate leanness and healthy aging: I learned it from bodybuilders who knew this decades before the nutrition and medical world figured it out.

If your body doesn't get the fuel it needs, it will begin the process of *catabolism:* breaking down muscle tissue and converting it into glucose, the body's ultimate fuel, so that it can continue to carry out your bodily functions. Not only does eating small, frequent meals prevent catabolism, but you will also feel less hungry throughout the day and will instinctively eat fewer calories. Best of all, you'll have the energy you need to perform better during your workouts and throughout the day, and you will drop body fat like never before.

You may also lower your cholesterol levels. In a study just reported in the *British Medical Journal*, it was shown that people who eat six or more times a day have cholesterol levels that are roughly 5 percent lower than those of less frequent eaters. According to the scientists, when you eat larger meals and go for longer periods of time between meals, insulin peaks at higher levels. High peaks of insulin alter fat and cholesterol metabolism—producing higher levels of cholesterol in your blood. Frequent small meals control insulin secretion and prevent these peaks: the result—lower levels of cholesterol. While a 5 percent reduction in cholesterol levels doesn't sound like much, it does have a large impact on your health, since it will reduce the risk of coronary artery disease by 10 percent.

The whole idea of eating more often to lose weight is one of the toughest concepts for me to get across to my patients. I know that it seems counterintuitive to suggest that you can lose weight by eating more often. I've got to admit, it took me a long time to believe that it works. But it really does. Once your body gets use to eating every three to four hours you become a fat-burning machine. Your body craves nutrients to keep its metabolic processes cranking along at top speed. When I eat one of my small 300-calorie meals, my body literally gets hot and my energy levels increase. The key is to not give it more calories than it needs at any one time.

When you eat frequent small meals you also avoid a common problem with most diets—caloric restriction. When people severely restrict their daily caloric intake, their body rapidly goes into starvation mode. The first thing that happens when you enter the starvation mode is that your basal metabolic rate begins to slow down. With severe caloric restriction your resting metabolic rate can drop by as much as 40 to 50 percent. Next, you begin metabolizing your own muscle tissue, converting it into glucose in order to preserve fat stores—that's right, all your hard-earned muscle starts disappearing. And, as if all of this isn't bad enough, the activity of fat-storing enzymes increases, and your fat-burning enzymes decrease, so that you become very efficient at storing body fat.

DON'T SKIP MEALS

Every overfat/obese man I have ever met has told me he doesn't eat breakfast. Skipping meals—especially breakfast—in order to limit calories is the number-one reason for failing to achieve lifelong leanness and muscularity. It is also the main cause for eating the wrong foods later in the day. Every time you miss a meal your blood sugar drops, increasing your hunger and cravings, which leads, at the very least, to overeating later in the day or, at the very worst, to eating the wrong foods. Poor control invariably means you will eat foods that are high in calories and low in nutrients—the very thing you are trying to avoid. Plan ahead so that you can always eat at scheduled mealtimes. It is absolutely an essential part of your transformation program.

Your appetite and cravings begin to skyrocket. If you don't have the willpower to resist these temptations, it won't be very long before lethargy, fatigue, and a total loss of desire to train take over and your entire program will be sabotaged. Sooner or later you, like everybody who follows a strict calorie and food-restricted diet, will "fall off the wagon" and "normal" eating or binge eating will take over. The result is always more fat and less muscle than you had when you started.

There is absolutely nothing that you can do to prevent this from happening except to never allow your caloric intake to drop below 1,200 to 1,500 calories each day. This will ensure a one- to two-pound weight loss per week, which the American College of Sports Medicine (ACSM) recommends as a safe level that ensures mostly fat loss. The more slowly you lose weight, the easier it is to hold on to your lean muscle mass and take the fat off, and the more likely it will be that you don't put it back on.

BILL TRICKED HIS BODY INTO LOSING WEIGHT

Bill is a 48-year-old surgeon who didn't realize that his extreme girth was a sign of disease. Over the past ten years, Bill hadn't been watching the scale, and instead was raiding the fridge whenever he felt stressed. Before he knew it, he was 30 pounds overweight, and his sexual function had decreased dramatically. He was having trouble getting out of bed each morning and felt as though he was losing his edge at work—constantly worried that younger surgeons would take over his practice.

When Bill came to see me, I first helped him identify his bad eating habits. I persuaded him to start a food diary and write down everything he ate and drank. The most important detail we uncovered was that Bill, like many men, was in the habit of skipping breakfast and not eating until several hours later. While a big lunch kept him from snacking throughout the day, he was inadvertently forcing his body into a "starvation mode" every morning. This meant that his body was storing nearly every calorie from lunch and dinner as body fat to get him through until lunch the next day. His body fat was not only collecting around his middle, it was slowing his metabolic rate for what his body perceived as an impending famine. In other words, his body was fighting to stay alive in a war that didn't really exist.

Once I rearranged Bill's daily eating routine, he started eating every three to four hours. His body was able to realize it wasn't starving, and it started burning its fat stores rather than storing calories as body fat. Six weeks later, Bill had lost 15 pounds and dropped from 34 percent body fat to 28 percent. Not only was he feeling and looking better, but his energy levels bounced back and his erectile function improved.

Keeping an accurate food diary is one of the most important indicators of the success of a fat-loss and strength-building program. When people don't keep track of what they eat, when they eat, and how much they eat, they invariably underestimate the volume of food, the number of calories, and the kinds of food they consume. A well-kept food diary will enable you to review, in the greatest of detail, your eating patterns and will allow you to make adjustments and choices that will keep you on track and assure you of continued success.

I think it is also very important to include in your diary a record of how you feel, both physically and emotionally, and monthly photos of you in a bathing suit (front, side, and back shots). As I said before, what you eat can have a profound effect on your moods, your energy levels, and the control you have over your eating. Everyone is different. Foods affect each of us in different ways, and the best way to discover how you react to a particular food is to keep an accurate record of what you eat and what it does to you. This will help you discover what *your* body really needs and wants and what it doesn't need or want. Most people go through their entire lives and never have a clue about how the foods they eat affect their emotional and physical lives and well-being.

Rule Two: Know Your Macronutrient Ratio

I have a simple rule that will help you balance each one of the five to six meals you'll be eating every day. Each meal's caloric makeup will consist of one-half to one part fat, two parts protein, and three parts healthy carbohydrates.

For example, if you are following the Basic Health Diet, and eating 1,800 calories per day, you'll eat 360 calories per meal for a total of 5 meals.

1. Fat—150 to 300 cal/day   or 30 to 60 cal/meal

2. Protein—600 cal/day   or 120 cal/meal

3. Carbohydrates—900 cal/day   or 180 cal/meal

Protein and carbs have 4 cal/gram and fat has 9 cal/gram. You can determine the number of grams of each nutrient group you should consume at any meal by dividing the calories per meal by 4 or 9.

For example: 1 serving of Fat—60 cal/9 = 6.6 gm of fat per meal.

PROTEINS BUILD MUSCLE

Protein and its amino acids are the building blocks of muscle and are an essential part of the human diet for the growth and repair of tissue. Adequate protein is necessary for optimizing hormones, increasing lean body mass, and decreasing body fat. High-quality proteins contain the most amino acids: Examples of quality protein are chicken or turkey, protein shakes, low-fat cottage cheese, lean meats, fish, soy products, and egg whites. Vegetarians and vegans need to make sure they eat plenty of high-protein vegetables such as beans, tempeh, soybeans, and tofu to meet their muscle-building needs.

A very convenient, practical, and efficient way to make sure you are getting enough high-quality protein without any added fat or cholesterol is by supplementing your diet with protein-containing nutritionals (such as protein powders, meal-replacement drinks, and sports bars). This is especially important for men who exercise, since an inadequate protein intake is related to the depletion of essential amino acids that occurs during intense training. In addition, high-quality proteins and essential amino acids have a positive influence on our hormonal and immune response to exercise, and they also enhance our ability to adapt to high-intensity training.

For years we thought that different types of proteins acted the same way within the body. However, a 1999 study, published in the *American Journal of Clinical Nutrition*, on sedentary overweight men (aged 51 to 69) with sarcopenia (muscle loss) cast doubt on this notion. The study divided the subjects into two groups: One ate meat, including beef, poultry, pork, and fish. The other group ate a lactoovovegetarian diet: only milk, eggs, and vegetables. Both groups participated in the same resistance-training programs. After 12 weeks both groups underwent extensive testing for strength and body composition changes. Muscle strength improved considerably in both groups to about the same degree. Changes in body composition, however, were very different. The meat eaters experienced gains in their fat-free mass characterized by muscle enlargement and a loss of body fat, while the vegetarians increased their percentage of body fat and decreased their muscle mass.

If you want to increase your muscle mass and get rid of body fat you need to get most of your protein from lean meat and beans, unless you are on the Heart Health Diet. The reason for this may relate to the effect a meat-eating diet has on a man's androgen hormone status and protein metabolism. Testosterone plays a key role in regulating and stimulating the synthesis of proteins—especially muscle protein.

Most authorities today believe that endurance athletes and bodybuilders require the most protein, and a very general recommendation now is that these people should consume 0.6 grams to 1 gram per pound of body weight. Consuming a slightly higher amount of protein won't hurt you, but very often you will see recommendations to consume much greater amounts of protein (up to 2 grams or more per pound of body weight). The consensus is that consuming extreme amounts of protein can lead to dehydration and a loss of calcium, and it also may put an increased load on your kidneys. In addition to all this, excess protein is often simply excreted or stored as fat, which doesn't help if you're trying to get stronger and leaner.

Now, if you're like me, the thought of counting out grams of protein for the rest of your life is a bit daunting. Luckily, I have a simpler, cleaner solution—the nutrition method in my Life Healthy Eating Plan provides about one gram of protein per pound of body weight daily, which falls right in the recommended range for muscle and strength building. You will be eating approximately 30 to 35 grams of protein with each of your small meals. Each serving size of protein is about the size and thickness of your palm.

HOW THE BODY REACTS TO PROTEIN

These are signals your body is sending to you about your current protein consumption:

- If you are usually hungry 1 to 2 hours after a meal, you are not eating enough healthy fat or protein.

- If you are hungry 3 to 4 hours after a meal, your protein intake is optimal.

- If you are not hungry for 5 to 7 hours after a meal, you ate too much protein.

THE RIGHT FATS KEEP YOU FEELING SATISFIED

Healthy types of dietary fat allow your body to feel satisfied after eating, build hormones, ensure the integrity of all your cell walls, insulate and protect your organs, and transport nutrients throughout your body. Eating fat is not problematic; eating the wrong *types* of fat is. Assessing the many types and forms of dietary fat can seem complicated, but ultimately, the bottom line is: The optimal types of fat are found in natural foods, such as fish, nuts, seeds, olives, and animal proteins. Dietary fats found in processed foods are *not* healthy.

KNOW YOUR FATS

The fats in your diet can contribute to early aging. It is therefore very important for you to have some basic knowledge about the difference between healthy fats and unhealthy fats so that you can make intelligent decisions.

SATURATED FATS

Saturated fats are solid at room temperature. Butter, cheese, and cream are all high in saturated fat, as is the fat on meat, and the so-called tropical oils (coconut, palm, and palm kernel oil). Saturated fats increase the amount of "bad" cholesterol (low-density lipoprotein, or LDL—remember, "L" equals lethal) in the blood, which can lead to atherosclerosis, heart disease, erectile dysfunction, and the restriction of blood flow. When saturated fats are incorporated into your cell membranes, the membranes tend to become rigid and less flexible, which in turn can affect their receptor mechanisms. This may explain why saturated fats are associated with insulin resistance and type 2 diabetes. In addition, diets high in animal fat are associated with colon cancer.

This form of fat has been clearly shown to be the key factor in causing coronary heart disease in a 25-year study involving seven countries. Saturated fats have recently been shown to interfere with athletic performance because they cause high insulin levels, leading to carbohydrate cravings, weight gain, impaired muscle growth, fatigue, and loss of endurance.

All of these adverse effects can be avoided simply by replacing saturated fats with "healthy fats"—monounsaturated fats. This will not only prevent the development of serious diseases but will improve your performance in and out of the gym.

CHOOSING PROTEIN SOURCES: FREE RANGE/ ORGANIC/GRASS-FED

Organic refers to the lack of chemicals present in the growing of a plant or raising of an animal. Free-range animal meats contain a better ratio of good to bad fats compared to traditionally raised animals that are fed grains to fatten them up faster. Grass contains omega-3 fatty acids, which have anti-inflammatory effects, whereas grains contain more omega-6 fatty acids, which have a proinflammatory effect. Nonorganic meats contain certain amounts of antibiotics and bovine growth hormone. Hormone-free animal and dairy products are recommended in my diet.

TRANS-FATTY ACIDS OR HYDROGENATED FATS

Hydrogenated (or partially hydrogenated) fats are liquid oils that have been artificially saturated with hydrogen to create a solid fat with a longer shelf life. Margarine and vegetable shortening are examples of this highly unnatural type of fat. The manufacturing process starts with healthy oils and ends up with a product that's bad for you.

Hydrogenated and partially hydrogenated fats not only are saturated, but also contain *trans-fatty acids,* a type of fatty acid that is not created in the body and is rarely found in nature. Trans-fatty acids are found in all fried foods, as well as in commercial brands of liquid oils, which are extracted using heat. They increase serum levels of "bad" cholesterol (LDL) and decrease the "good" cholesterol (high-density lipoprotein, or HDL—remember, "H" equals healthy), and are heavily associated with coronary heart disease. They have been shown to adversely affect metabolic processes in heart tissue. Trans-fatty acids are also incorporated into cell membranes even though they are not normal components of human tissue. When this occurs, they interfere with the function of cell membranes, making cells less flexible and blocking natural biochemical pathways.

Hydrogenated and partially hydrogenated oils are used extensively in commercially prepared foods, including peanut butter, mayonnaise, baked goods, margarine, and chocolate. If you are serious about cutting back on your fat intake, especially harmful fats, you'll need to make a point of staying away from these very bad fat sources.

MONOUNSATURATED FATTY ACIDS

Monounsaturated fats are usually liquid at room temperature, but may solidify in the refrigerator. Monounsaturated fats contain a high proportion of oleic acid, a fatty acid that can be synthesized by all mammals, including humans. Monounsaturated oils include olive oil, peanut oil, avocado oil, and canola oil. Because they aren't harmful, they can be considered healthful. Long-term consumption of these oils (especially olive oil) in several southern European countries is associated with low overall mortality rates and low incidence of coronary heart disease. Olive oil is 72 percent monounsaturated; canola oil (actually extracted from rapeseed) is 65 percent monounsaturated; and peanut oil is 48 percent monounsaturated. Canola and peanut oils are likely to contain chemical residues from the way the plants were raised. Avocado oil is extremely expensive. Your best choices are olive oil—preferably cold-pressed and unrefined ("extra-virgin")—and avocados.

POLYUNSATURATED FATTY ACIDS

Safflower, sunflower, corn, sesame, and soy oils are all polyunsaturated fatty acids (PUFAs). Even though they are cholesterol free and low in saturated fat, these oils can still cause problems by creating oxidation products that form free radicals that damage DNA, alter cell membranes, and promote cancer. The breakdown of polyunsaturated fatty acids produces more oxidants than the breakdown of other types of fats. This is because of the multiple double bonds found in polyunsaturated fats. Each double bond provides an opportunity for oxidation. The more polyunsaturated an oil is, the more double bonds it has, and the more potential there is for free-radical formation. Safflower oil is the most unsaturated vegetable oil, and as such can cause significant immune suppression. This is surprising news to many consumers who were told that polyunsaturated oils were part of a healthy diet.

ESSENTIAL FATTY ACIDS

Omega-3 and omega-6 fatty acids are both essential fatty acids that the body cannot make, so it is up to us to make sure we eat foods that contain them. Many Americans (especially those who follow low-fat diets) suffer from an essential fatty acid deficiency. We now know that this deficiency is detrimental to our physical and mental well-being, causing serious diseases, including atherosclerosis (plugging of arteries), strokes, coronary heart disease, erratic heart-beats leading to sudden cardiac death, rheumatoid and degenerative arthritis, skin problems including wrinkles, loss of vision, and degenerative brain diseases.

There are three main types of omega-3 fats—EPA (eicosapentaenoic acid), DHA (doco-sahexaenoic acid), and ALA (alpha-linolenic acid). EPA and DHA are the "marine" omega-3s found in fish. ALA is found mostly in plant oils. These essential fatty acids are required to make a family of hormones called eicosanoids—substances that are potent mediators of many biochemical functions that play a critical role in coordinating a number of physiological functions such as blood clotting, blood pressure, blood vessel dilation, heart rate, heart rhythm, muscle and bone growth, and immune response.

Most authorities believe that EPA and DHA are the omega-3 fats that play the greatest role in promoting health and preventing disease. ALA (found in flaxseed) is an indirect source of EPA and DHA. However, we can convert only less than 15 percent of ALA into EPA and DHA, so most experts think flaxseed is a poor way to get adequate amounts of EPA and DHA.

Getting the right amounts of good fats was easier in the past, because foods contained the right ratios of omega-6 to omega-3 fatty acids. Unfortunately, omega-3 fatty acids are not nearly as plentiful in the foods we eat today, because food companies have deliberately destroyed them in order to increase the shelf life of their products. The meat from today's cows and chickens has much less omega-3 fatty acid since these animals are now fed processed grains low in omega-3s instead of wild plants and seeds, which are naturally high in these fats. As a result, we now consume one-sixth the amount of omega-3 fatty acids that our ancestors did, which has drastically increased our ratio

MARGARINE VERSUS BUTTER

Actually, olive oil is a better choice than either margarine or butter, but if you must choose between a small amount of butter and a small amount of margarine, choose butter. Margarine can contain up to 30 percent trans-fatty acids, while butter, although it is a saturated fat, is a more natural product. Benecol and Smart Balance are also healthy options.

By choosing olive oil instead of butter or margarine, you avoid the hazards of saturated fat and you also avoid the immune-suppressing effects of the more harmful trans-fatty acids.

CHOOSE PROTEIN PACKED WITH THE RIGHT FAT

Omega-3 eggs are laid by chickens that have been fed flaxseeds. The eggs actually contain more omega-3 fatty acids, a healthy essential fat, and less saturated fat than those laid by grain/corn-fed chickens.

of omega-6s to omega-3s to 20 to 1. The current ratio dramatically interferes with many of the key functions of essential fatty acids, including the synthesis of prostaglandin hormones—hormones that govern all cell growth, blood clotting, and our immune function. This imbalance may promote heart disease, obesity, diabetes, and some cancers.

On the Life Plan, your goal is to achieve a ratio of less than 4 omega-6s to 1 omega-3s. The best way to do this is to avoid foods fried in vegetable oils, such as corn and safflower, and eliminate processed foods, which contain large amounts of omega-6s. At the same time, you will increase the amount of omega-3s in your diet by eating green leafy vegetables and more oily fish, such as sardines, herring, bluefish, shrimp, flounder, mackerel, wild salmon, and swordfish. For those who don't like fish, fish oil supplements are now an option: You should take 3 to 4 grams per day. Cooking with canola oil instead of vegetable oil also helps.

KEVIN AVOIDED ALL FATS AND DRIED OUT

Kevin was a 55-year-old photographer with coronary artery disease. He had read about the low-fat, high-complex-carbohydrate diet recommended by Dean Ornish, M.D., and took it to an extreme. He avoided *all* fats. Unfortunately, Kevin developed dry skin, constipation, increased thirst, brittle nails, and dry hair—all signs of essential fatty acid deficiency.

After I taught Kevin how to include healthy fats in his diet and he added essential fatty acid supplements to his program, his symptoms resolved without compromising his heart condition—and he felt a whole lot better.

THE RIGHT CARBS ENERGIZE YOUR WORKOUTS; THE WRONG CARBS WILL KILL YOU

Over the last 10 to 20 years we have been convinced by the American Heart Association, USDA Food Pyramid, and the food manufacturers that high-carbohydrate/low-fat diets are the way to eat if we want to avoid heart disease and achieve ultimate health. We have all been led to believe that fats are bad and carbohydrates in any form are okay when it comes to healthy eating. We have actually been given license to eat any and all carbs with little or no regard to whether they are the healthy types (vegetables and fruits) or the unhealthy, highly processed types produced by the profit-motivated food manufacturers.

Vegetables and most fruits are healthy carbohydrates because they are digested very slowly and enter our bloodstream in small amounts, gently and gradually increasing our blood sugars. Man-made carbohydrates, on the other hand, come from grains that undergo processing that removes most of their natural fiber and nutrients, making them easily digestible and rapidly assimilated by our bodies. These carbohydrates have very high glycemic indexes (a measure of how fast a particular food will raise your blood sugar), and they mainline sugar into our bloodstream, pushing blood sugars and insulin levels sky-high, causing subsequent huge drops in blood sugars. As our blood sugars fall, hunger returns, cravings rapidly follow, and compulsive, uncontrolled eating takes over. This vicious cycle is replayed countless times, day in and day out, throughout America by most of us who have bought into the high-carb/low-fat mind-set.

UNDERSTANDING THE GLYCEMIC INDEX

The glycemic index determines how fast a particular food will raise your blood sugar. Glucose forms the base number of the index because it's the second-fastest sugar to get into your bloodstream—maltose is the fastest. Glucose is given a value of 100, and other carbohydrates are given values relative to glucose depending on how fast they get into your blood—the lower the index the longer it takes. Diabetics have successfully used the glycemic index for many years to help control their blood sugars. Recently, people who have wanted to lose weight and prevent cravings have used this index. The idea is that when blood sugar and insulin levels are kept low, your body is much less likely to convert sugars to body fat, and food cravings are reduced or even eliminated altogether. This has worked very well for me, and I recommend it to all of you as another tool that can be used to get lean and stay lean.

You can find a glycemic index list of some of the common foods we eat on my website, www.drlife.com. Foods that have a high index (greater than 60) include ice cream, white breads, all white flour products, bagels, white potatoes, bananas, raisins, potato chips, alcoholic beverages, white rice, and pastas made with white flour.

Low-glycemic-index foods (under 45) include most fruits and vegetables, whole wheat or whole grain foods, regular oatmeal, sugar-free peanut butter, high-fiber sugar-free cereals, yams, brown rice, sugar-free dairy products, grains, legumes (with the exception of baked beans and fava beans), new potatoes, nuts, and most vegetables.

The evidence is overwhelming that the overfat/obesity and type 2 diabetes epidemics are a direct result of our obsession with high-glycemic carbohydrates. It is absolutely critical that the carbohydrates you eat be mostly those with a low glycemic index to ensure the maintenance of low levels of blood sugar and insulin. We should limit our intake of high-glycemic carbs to only immediately before or immediately after a high-intensity weight-training workout. This will shuttle muscle-building nutrients quickly into muscle tissue and promote growth and strength.

CARBOHYDRATES AND FOOD ADDICTION

Unfortunately, carbohydrates now form the bulk of our diets. Seventy-five percent of all Americans overreact to carbohydrates and produce too much insulin in their bodies. This causes marked fluctuations in blood sugars and higher-than-normal baseline levels of insulin, which, over time, can create a dependency on sugar and highly processed carbohydrates, leading ultimately to more fatness and obesity along with serious health consequences.

In spite of all this, our love for sweets and processed carbohydrates continues to escalate. We eat an average of 20 teaspoons of sugar every day. That's 320 calories daily, or 117,000 calories a year, which our bodies convert into 33 pounds of fat. And this doesn't include the natural sugars found in fruits, vegetables, and milk—it's just the sugar that is added to our foods. It includes white, raw, brown, or cane sugar; corn syrup or high-fructose corn syrup; molasses, honey, or sorghum syrup; and fruit juice concentrate. No matter what it is called, it's all the same—just plain old white table sugar, which has 4 calories per gram and no other nutrients.

Recent studies done at the University of Wisconsin have demonstrated that fat alone, or the combination of fat with sugar or salt, has a powerful neurochemical effect on the brain, causing it to release certain natural chemicals similar to drugs like heroin and morphine that activate pleasure centers and promote addiction. Dr. Ann Kelly, a professor of psychiatry and neuroscience and the senior author of the study, believes it is the fat that is the primary addicting culprit—especially when it is combined with sugar or salt.

This study, which strongly suggests that fast food is addictive, is expected to be the basis of a number of obesity lawsuits filed against the fast-food industry. In fact, lawyer John Banzhaf III, famous for his battles against the tobacco industry, has already used some of Dr. Kelly's research as a foundation for lawsuits he is threatening to bring against six fast-food giants (McDonald's, Burger King, Wendy's, Taco Bell, Pizza Hut, and Kentucky Fried Chicken).

An ultra-low-carbohydrate eating plan is the only way I know to beat carbohydrate addiction. My plan is easy to follow, and I can personally confirm that your hunger will be well controlled and your food cravings and compulsive eating will come to a rapid stop. On this plan you will limit your intake of all carbs to less than 30 grams a day, and replace the carbohydrates you have eliminated with high-quality protein containing low amounts of saturated fat.

My Life Plan diet differs significantly from Dr. Atkins's low-carb diet, because he promoted (actually encouraged) the consumption of unhealthy saturated fats found in red meats, bacon, and dairy products, while I believe that these fats need to be avoided, since they are proven to cause heart disease. Instead, you will be replacing unhealthy fats with the disease-fighting essential fatty acids and monounsaturated fats I mentioned above. The reason this very-low-carb diet does such a great job in controlling eating and cravings is that it rapidly achieves control over blood sugars and insulin levels and thereby prevents the vicious cycle of hyperinsulinism (high insulin levels) followed by low blood sugar levels—the root cause of cravings and addiction to sugar and processed carbohydrates.

Within a few days after you start this approach, your cravings for sweets, breads, pastas, and bagels will begin to subside. After one week, the cravings will completely disappear and you will notice that your energy levels and endurance dramatically increase. Stay on it for a month and then gradually begin adding healthy carbohydrates (low-glycemic-index fruits and vegetables) back to your diet.

HIGH-FIBER FOODS ARE THE BEST CARBOHYDRATES

Fiber is vitally important—especially if you want to lose fat without jeopardizing your muscle mass and, at the same time, improve your overall health. On average, American men consume around 10 grams to 12 grams per day, and the recommended intake is 25 grams to 50 grams per day—preferably around 35 grams. In a major study published in the *Journal of the American Heart Association* in October 1999, it was shown that a high intake of fiber reduces not only obesity, but also reduces high blood pressure, other heart disease risk factors, and the risk of many cancers. Some experts even believe fiber plays a greater role in determining heart disease risk than total or saturated fat intake.

Dietary fiber does all of this by remaining mostly undigested in your gastrointestinal tract. This provides bulk to the foods you eat so that undigested food stays in the stomach longer, making you feel fuller and delaying hunger and cravings. Once the food reaches your intestines, it moves along at a faster rate, which slows the release of carbohydrates and cholesterol-raising fats into your bloodstream. Since sugars are slowly absorbed rather than mainlined into your bloodstream, blood sugar levels remain well controlled, and insulin secretion is reduced. Many experts now believe fiber's effect on blood sugar levels is the main reason for its "fat-fighting" properties and other health benefits.

Because fiber makes you feel full, you eat much less without even thinking about it. This was really brought to light in a recent study from Penn State that showed how people eat about the same *weight* of food on a daily basis. In other words, it is not the total number of calories consumed that controls how much you eat; instead, it's the volume or weight of the food that you eat that determines when you think you've have had enough. When you eat high-fiber foods, you consume a higher volume or weight of food with fewer calories—and you won't feel the least bit deprived.

The best fiber sources include whole natural foods such as fruits, vegetables, whole grains, and legumes. Avoid processed foods at all costs. Processed foods have had their fiber (along with many nutrients) removed, but not the calories, which will keep insulin levels high and add inches to your spare tire.

CARBOHYDRATE SENSITIVITY

Carbohydrate sensitivity is a term that researchers use to describe a volatile increase in blood sugar as a result of eating carbohydrates (especially those with a high glycemic index, such as the cookies and white bread you crave). As blood sugars rise, carbohydrate-sensitive individuals have very sensitive pancreatic tissue that overreacts and produces excessive amounts of insulin—rapidly driving their blood sugars down. As blood sugars plummet, extreme hunger and cravings, mostly for sweets, take over and this vicious cycle is repeated. Over time this can progress to full-blown insulin resistance syndrome, resulting in diabetes and serious blood vessel disease, hypertension, and premature death.

As many as 75 percent of overweight individuals are thought to be carbohydrate sensitive. Worse, as people with carbohydrate sensitivity age, their sensitivity also increases, and many prominent authorities now believe that this condition can progress to an actual chemical addiction similar to that seen with alcohol, nicotine, and drugs. They recommend that carbohydrate sensitivity be treated very much like these addictions—with abstinence.

The best way to determine if you are carbohydrate sensitive and, if so, to what degree, is by writing down in your food journal your reaction (both physical and emotional) to the foods you eat. This will enable you to "listen" to what your body is "telling" you, and it won't take long before you know which foods affect you the most.

WATER: DRINK HALF YOUR BODY WEIGHT IN OUNCES DAILY

Water is your most important nutrient. You can live only three days without it, and it is involved in every metabolic reaction in your body. Yet most of us don't drink enough. When we are properly hydrated our heart and blood vessels work much better, along with all of our other bodily functions—we think better, our strength and endurance are better, we feel better, we are healthier, and we will live longer. Adequate hydration has the added benefit of helping us eat less by giving us a satisfied feeling—a key ingredient to achieving and maintaining a lean, healthy lifestyle.

In one study from Berlin's Franz-Volhard Clinical Research Center, Michael Boschmann, M.D., and his colleagues tracked energy expenditures among seven men and seven women who were healthy and not overweight. After drinking approximately 17 ounces of water, the subjects' metabolic rates (the rate at which calories are burned) increased by 30 percent. The increases began within 10 minutes and reached a maximum after 30 to 40 minutes. The study also showed that the increase in metabolic rate differed in men and women. In men, extra water caused them to burn more fat, which fueled the increase in metabolism, whereas in women the additional water increased their breakdown of carbohydrates, which increased their metabolism. The researchers found that up to 40 percent of the increase in calorie burning was caused by the body's attempt to heat the ingested water. It appears from this study that the colder the water is, the better. A 2002 study published in the *American Journal of Epidemiology* found that drinking five or more glasses of water a day reduced the risk of a fatal heart attack by about 50 percent.

So there you have it, gentlemen: More water translates into more fat burned. Over the course of a year, if you can increase your water consumption to 1.5 liters a day, you will burn an extra 17,400 calories, for a weight loss of approximately five pounds.

In his book *The Blood Thinner Cure,* Dr. Kenneth R. Kensey wrote that most of us go through life in a dehydrated state because we rely on our sensation of thirst as our guide for water consumption. He states that by the time we are thirsty, we are already dehydrated and our blood is too thick, which may be one primary cause of hardening of the arteries, heart attacks, and strokes. I'm not sure I'd go that far, but I do know that a lack of water is the major reason for daytime fatigue. Even mild dehydration will slow your metabolism by as much as 3 percent. A mere 2 percent drop in body water can trigger fuzzy short-term memory, trouble with basic math, and difficulty focusing on the computer screen or on a printed page.

THE BEST PROCESSED FOOD CHOICES

- Packaged foods that are minimally processed with the most natural ingredients.

- Whole grains over whole wheat.

- Natural peanut butter: It's a great source of essential fatty acids, while processed peanut butter is loaded with sugar and hydrogenated oil.

- Low-fat dairy instead of fat-free: You need some of dairy's good fat, and fat-free products are usually supplemented with sugar to make them tastier.

- Brown rice and natural oatmeal over "instant" varieties: They have lower glycemic indexes.

Your ability to exercise at full capacity is directly dependent on adequate hydration. If you are as little as 1 percent dehydrated (1.5 pounds in a 150-pound person), all body functions suffer, and you will have a 10 percent decrease in your aerobic capacity. To make sure you're adequately hydrated, you should try to drink half an ounce of fluid per pound of body weight daily.

You'll be able to accomplish this by drinking small amounts of water throughout the day. For example, drink 1 tall glassful before you have your first cup of coffee in the morning and drink 1 to 2 cups of water 30 minutes before you exercise. Drink a half cup every 15 minutes during exercise and 1.5 cups to 3 cups over a one- to two-hour period after you finish exercising. Some people find it easier to keep a refillable bottle of water with them throughout the day. When I really focus on dropping body fat and training hard, I have a one-gallon jug of water that I carry around, and I try to consume most of it every day. Most people have no idea how much consuming adequate amounts of water can help them drop body fat and improve their performance. If you want to get really lean and improve your mental and physical performance, I challenge you to drink close to a gallon of water every day. You will be amazed at how much it helps. The best way to tell that you are getting enough fluids is that you should have to make frequent trips to the bathroom, and your urine will be clear, except for when you first go in the morning.

To mix things up, you can take your water in the form of sparkling water, tea, or coffee. A few squirts of lemon juice really help make water easier to drink.

MODERATE YOUR ALCOHOL INTAKE

Alcohol is a very concentrated source of calories (7 calories per gram) and, when it enters your bloodstream, your liver must reduce or stop its metabolism of fats and carbohydrates and many of its other vital functions in order to process it. This dramatically interferes with your successful exercise program by causing a buildup of fat in your liver, a decrease in glycogen (master fuel) formation in your liver and muscles, and an interference with niacin, thiamine, and B vitamins use—all essential for energy production and good health.

In addition, alcohol will stimulate your appetite (carbohydrate-sensitive people very often crave sweets when they drink), make it much harder to exercise, and act as a diuretic, causing you to lose precious water—all of which will sabotage your efforts to get lean, muscular, and healthy. My advice—use very little or none at all. If you want to see your six-pack abs, then you really need to give up alcohol.

The late coach John Wooden's adage, "If you fail to plan, you plan to fail, " holds very true in basketball and in other sports, but it is also very true when it comes to acheiving success with your exercise and nutrition program. When you wake up in the morning and are ready to start your day, think through where you are going to be eating, and how you will be able to access the food you need for five to six healthy meals. This might mean preparing meals in advance and taking them with you so that you don't find yourself hungry and trapped, pulling into a fast-food restaurant and eating a high-calorie, high-fat, low-nutrition meal.

Here are some of my best planning tips:

1. Cook enough protein and veggies to have meals ready in the fridge for several days. This is a huge time saver!

2. Always pack lunches and snacks to take with you.

3. Always have meal replacement bars and/or shakes on hand.

4. Plan according to your day's activities—bigger, higher-carb meals before a workout, smaller meals before a nap or watching TV.

5. Always carry water with you—a no-calorie way to fill yourself up between meals.

Making It Work

In the next chapter, you will decide which level of diet you want to enter, based on your current health and your weight loss goals. All three levels of diet are based on the rules and lessons presented in this chapter. In addition, here are some key rules I try to follow daily that really help me stay on track. Try them out and I think you will agree that they can play an essential role in helping you achieve your ultimate goals of leanness, energy, muscularity, and great health.

1. Make a list of the reasons you want to lose body fat and keep it off forever. Laminate it, carry it with you, and refer to it frequently.

2. Avoid buffets and other places where there are many food choices—the more food choices you have the more you will eat too much of the wrong foods.

3. No finger foods—ever.

4. Don't eat unless you are sitting at a table.

5. Avoid eating fast. Savor every bite. Try to spend 15 to 20 minutes eating each and every meal.

6. Avoid high-glycemic fruits (bananas, kiwis, pineapples, papayas, mangoes, honeydew melons, watermelons, cantaloupes, raisins) and all fruit juices.

7. Don't eat for at least two hours before you go to bed.

8. If you get a craving, avoid eating for at least 15 minutes—cravings invariably disappear by that time.

9. If you must have dairy, then go for low-fat or soy cheeses.

10. For snacks, have a protein shake, apple with low-fat cheese, orange with handful of almonds, or celery or carrots with low-fat cheese.

CHAPTER 3

The Life Plan Diets

I have devised three simple nutritional plans that create a stepped dieting approach toward a goal of completely clean eating. Each diet promotes health and youthful aging. Depending on your current health and fitness level, you can enter into any one of these plans at any point, and upgrade from one to the next. Obviously, the more limiting diets will achieve the best and fastest results.

Everyone should start with the Basic Health Diet and stick with it for at least three weeks. You will know if the diet is working by two important measurements: the scale, and your abdominal girth. By the end of three weeks, you should have lost at least five pounds and dropped at least half an inch from your abdomen, as measured in Chapter 2.

If you enjoy the diet, you can stay on this level forever. However, if you want faster results, move to the next level: the Fat-Burning Diet. The Fat-Burning Diet is more rigorous, but it is absolutely the best way I know to get rid of body fat. Like Basic Health, you can stay on this diet forever or until you are under 15 percent body fat.

If you still want to increase your weight loss to below 10 percent body fat or if you have already been diagnosed with a heart condition, have a stent, or have had bypass surgery, high blood pressure, or other vasculature problems, move to the final level: Heart Health. Your goal should be to follow the Heart Health Diet as closely as possible forever. This is a completely vegan diet that combines low-glycemic eating with a low-fat diet so that you can start reversing blood vessel disease. Moreover, if you are having problems with your sexual health, this is the diet to follow.

A Word about Protein Shakes

You'll see in the following meal plans that I'm a big fan of protein shakes. When combined with fruit, they help my body recover from aggressive exercise by restoring muscle glycogen. They also can contribute to muscle repair.

I usually drink protein shakes twice a day: once in the morning after my morning workout, then a plain chocolate casein protein shake (no fruit) about 30 minutes before bed. Casein is a type of protein that is found in milk. Casein is known to have a slow absorption rate, allowing the amino acids in the protein shake to enter the bloodstream slowly. This keeps you feeling full and satisfied for a longer period of time. Casein is an excellent source of protein to consume before bedtime, which usually precedes the longest interval of time between meals, because it really helps prevent "nighttime munchies."

Shakes use a variety of protein sources, such as whey, casein, egg, soy, and milk. These sources may affect your body differently. I've found both whey and casein to be smart choices. Because casein is absorbed slowly, it prevents nighttime munchies, and I can go to sleep much faster without obsessing about foods in the refrigerator.

COOKING WITH PROTEIN POWDERS

When I'm bored with drinking protein shakes, I sometimes add protein powder to my oatmeal in the morning. Heating or cooking the powder unwinds the string of amino acids in the protein molecule and breaks it into smaller pieces. In other words, it starts the digestive process and makes it easier for you to process the amino acids and get them into your bloodstream faster.

The only time I promote eating a high-glycemic carb is within an hour after aggressive resistance training leading to muscle failure. Muscle failure is the physical point of exhaustion, when it is physically impossible to perform another repetition of a particular exercise. I throw a banana into my 8- to 10-ounce chocolate protein shake to bump up blood sugars and insulin levels, which will drive amino acids into the muscle tissue. That helps increase your amount of muscle tissue and strength.

However, don't confuse muscle failure with mental failure. If you're just too tired to exercise, you can't have that banana!

BENEFITS OF WHEY PROTEIN SHAKES

- Absorbs quickly

- Found in milk

- Digests quickly

- Excellent supplement after aggressive training

BENEFITS OF CASEIN PROTEIN SHAKES

- Absorbs slowly

- Key protein in milk

- Digests slowly

- Excellent supplement before bed—helps you sleep

Quick Shopping List for Basic Health and Fat-Burning Diets

Here are some of the foods you'll need on hand no matter which of these diet levels you begin with:

- Avocados

- Chicken or turkey breasts

- Fresh fruits

- Fresh or flash-frozen fish: salmon, steelhead trout, tuna, sardines (not canned), or mackerel

- Fresh vegetables

- High-fiber cereal

- Low-fat dairy cheeses and yogurts

- Low-fat vinaigrette salad dressing

- Olive oil, canola oil

- Omega-3 eggs

- Skim milk or soy milk

- Turkey jerky

- Whole grain bread with a minimum of 3 grams of fiber per slice

- Yams

RAFAEL MEDINA

"Dr. Life allowed me to completely reinvent myself. I was at a point in my life where I had gained over 25 pounds and I had lost all my drive and motivation. After meeting Dr. Life I was able to wake up every day with the motivation to follow an intense workout regimen and make healthier dietary decisions. Just two years later I've lost 23.7 pounds of body fat and gained 21 pounds of muscle. I feel like I'm in my 20s again and I'm in the best shape of my life!

"Thanks, Dr. Life!"

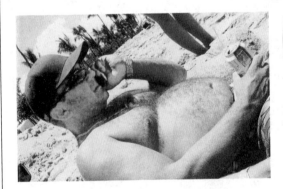

The Basic Health Diet

The Basic Health Diet is a low-glycemic, insulin-control diet designed to reduce blood pressure and cardiovascular disease while improving overall health and body composition. It focuses on natural foods, not just lower-glycemic fruits and vegetables.

My Food Pyramid can help you understand my low-glycemic Basic Health Diet.

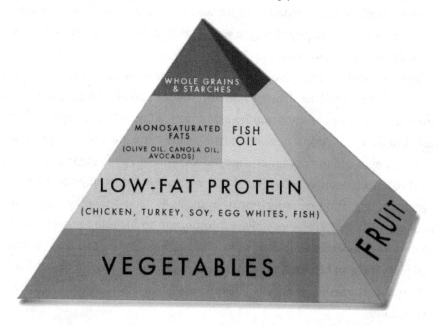

Dr. Life's Food Pyramid for the Basic Health Diet

The USDA's Food Pyramid ignores the impact certain foods have on blood sugar, disregards insulin control, and has contributed to our national obesity epidemic. My version creates a much better environment for your body to control blood sugar levels and insulin production, reducing and/or preventing your risk for silent inflammation. It's the starting point for optimized health and better body composition. Low-fat protein—chicken, turkey, fish, soy, lean meat, low-fat diary, and eggs—works synergistically with fruit and veggies to keep insulin levels down. You'll notice there are whole grains and complex carbohydrate starches, but few of them. Limiting whole grains delivers the best opportunity for reduced disease risk. So focus on small amounts of rolled oats, pumpernickel, rye, whole wheat, quinoa, brown rice, and other whole grain options. This is also different from the popular Mediterranean Diet, which is tilted on the grain-starch side and elevates blood sugars and insulin levels. My pyramid also uses fats in moderation, and limits those fats to fish oil and monounsaturated fats.

When you are following the Basic Health Diet, you will be having five or six meals a day at three- to four-hour intervals. The recipes and menu suggestions for these healthy food choices can be easily prepared by steaming, grilling, or stir-frying with small amounts of oil. Follow this rotation for one week and then repeat. You can also mix up the days, but try to keep the meals together. At the end of the chapter, there are simple recipes that you can substitute as well if you prefer to cook your meals once a week, as I do.

If you are currently a vegetarian, you will need to make some changes to this diet or simply go to my Heart Health Diet. However, many strict vegans are dangerously low in energy-creating nutrients, protein, essential amino acids, iron, vitamin B12, calcium, vitamin D, and zinc. The risk of these nutritional deficiencies is even greater while you are following an intense muscle- and strength-building program, like the one you will be following in this plan.

Because of this, I strongly recommend that vegetarians, especially vegans, take great care in planning, selecting, and preparing nutritious meals to make sure they are getting adequate amounts of essential nutrients. Not only is it important to include the essential micronutrients (vitamins and minerals) and macronutrients (carbohydrates, fats, and proteins) in your nutritional plan, it is also helpful if each meal consists of one portion of carbohydrate and one portion of protein. A portion of each can be measured against the size of a clenched fist or the palm of your hand.

PREPARING MEATS AND VEGETABLES

The way you prepare vegetables significantly affects their nutrient levels. Spinach, carrots, and tomatoes actually have higher antioxidant levels when they are heated. But in most cases, heat and water strip away valuable nutrients, including vitamins and disease-fighting phytochemicals. It's best to avoid cooking vegetables with water that is later discarded. If your vegetables are cooked in stews and soups, then the nutrients are retained.

Try to eat as many of your vegetables raw (well washed) as you can. If you like them cooked, the best way to maximize their nutrient content is by using a microwave, pressure cooker, or steamer.

Animal proteins should always be thoroughly cooked. There are many infectious diseases you can get from raw poultry, fish, eggs, and meats. Some of the infections can actually make you "ICU sick, " with IVs, a Foley catheter, an arterial line, and sometimes even a respirator. Obviously, this will not be good for your training program.

Eggs Are Never a Bad Protein Choice

Egg yolks have gotten a bad rap over the last several years, and this is because they have fairly high levels of saturated fat and cholesterol, which are thought to contribute to heart disease. Recently we have learned that egg yolks can be an excellent source of omega-3 fatty acids, which may actually reduce the risk for heart and blood vessel disease as well as high blood pressure, arthritis, cancer, and diabetes.

However, most of the eggs sold in U.S. grocery stores do not contain much omega-3. The reason is that these eggs come from factory-farmed chickens, which are kept in cages and fed grains that produce little omega-3. Eggs produced by organically fed, free-range chickens have a much higher content of omega-3 fatty acids: This is one case where I believe organic is worth the extra money. And keep in mind that the effects of egg yolks on human cholesterol levels is greatly overshadowed by the large amounts of dietary saturated fat most Americans get from butter, cheese, cream, red meat, and baked goods.

Even if you do eat the best eggs, you should still be somewhat careful about how many yolks you eat, since their cholesterol content may increase your cholesterol level. Most people can eat one egg yolk a day without any problem. And while you may want to minimize your consumption of egg yolks, you most definitely don't want to avoid the whites. They're a great source of high-quality, muscle-building protein.

Basic Health Diet

Many of these meals are self-explanatory and require no cooking and little preparation: in other words, they are perfectly suited for men like me. Others require very rudimentary cooking skills, like chopping, baking, boiling, or broiling. Most of these meals can be prepared in a microwave oven as well. Just complete the instructions that precede the ingredients list to create a satisfying and easy-to-prepare single dish.

While you can repeat days if you find some more appealing than others, don't swap out individual meals. Otherwise, your numbers will be off.

BASIC HEALTH DIET

Food		Calories	Fat Grams	Protein Grams	Carb Grams
MEAL #1: Combine oats and milk in a large microwave-safe dish. Cook in microwave oven on high for 3 minutes or until oatmeal is thoroughly cooked to the consistency you prefer—more time may be needed. Top with blueberries. In a separate lightly oiled pan, scramble the egg whites and serve on the side.					
Starch	½ cup rolled oats	303	5.4	13.2	51.7
Very lean protein	5 egg whites	86	0.3	18	0
Low-fat milk	½ cup 1% milk	53	1.2	4.3	6.1
Fruit	2.4 oz blueberries	39	0.2	0.5	9.9
MEAL #2					
Fruit	1 large (7.9 oz) apple	116	0.4	0.6	30.8
Very lean protein	1 scoop whey protein drink	110	0.75	22	0.5
MEAL #3: Combine all the ingredients (except for the soup) on a single plate to create a salad.					
Very lean protein	4 oz canned tuna (in water, not oil)	122	1.2	26.5	0
Vegetable	2 cups shredded lettuce	32	0.6	6	2.4
Vegetable	½ cup tomato	16	0.2	0.8	3.5
Vegetable	½ cup cucumber	7	0.1	0.3	1.3
Vegetable	1 oz chopped red onion	12	0.1	0.3	2.9
Monounsaturated	2 oz olives	82	8.7	0.6	2.2

Food		Calories	Fat Grams	Protein Grams	Carb Grams
Polyunsaturated	2 tbs fat-free Italian dressing	13	0.3	0.3	2.5
Soup/Starch	1.5 cup "Not So Portuguese" kale soup	102	2	3	18
MEAL #4					
Vegetable	2 stalks celery	5	0.1	2	1.2
Monounsaturated	2 tbs natural reduced-fat peanut butter	200	12	9	12
Fruit	1 large (7.4 oz) pear	121	0.8	0.8	32.4
MEAL #5					
Very lean protein	4 oz 96% lean beef, broiled	185	6.7	29.2	0
Starch	5 oz baked or microwaved yam	164	0.1	2.1	39.1
Vegetable	8 asparagus spears	26	0.2	1.4	2.5
Vegetable	5 oz roasted red peppers	51	0	0	5.1
TOTAL		1827.95	41.3	140.9	224.1

DAY 2

Food		Calories	Fat Grams	Protein Grams	Carb Grams
MEAL #1: Combine ingredients in a single bowl.					
Very lean protein	1 cup low-fat cottage cheese 1%	81	1.1	14	3.1
Fruit	½ cup raspberries	32	0.4	0.7	7.3
Starch	½ cup low-fat granola	195	3	4	38
MEAL #2					
Fruit	1 cup cherries	194	0.6	2.2	49.2
Medium-fat protein	2 pieces string cheese	120	5	14	1
MEAL #3					
Very lean protein	6 oz shrimp, boiled	168	1.8	35.5	0
Vegetable	4 tbs salsa	20	0	0	5
Vegetable	3 cups mixed green salad	20	0	1	3
Monounsaturated	2 oz avocado	91	8.3	4.8	1.1
Starch	8 oz baked or microwaved yam	263	0.2	3.4	62.7

Food		Calories	Fat Grams	Protein Grams	Carb Grams
MEAL #4					
Very lean protein	1 oz nitrate-free turkey jerky	101.5	1	19.25	1
Fruit	1 large (7.4 oz) pear	121	0.2	0.8	32.4
MEAL #5: Combine pine nuts and vegetables to cooked rice before eating.					
Very lean protein	4 oz flounder, broiled	132	1.7	27.3	0
Monounsaturated	1 tbs extra-virgin olive oil (for coating the fish before broiling)	120	14	0	0
Monounsaturated	20 pine nuts (about .2 oz)	11	1.2	0.2	0.2
Vegetable	1 cup steamed broccoli	55	0.6	3.7	11.2
Vegetable	1 cup(2.5 oz) steamed bok choy	9	0.1	1	1.5
Starch	1 cup cooked wild rice	83	0.25	3.25	17.45
TOTAL		1831.65	39.45	135.1	234.15

DAY 3

Food		Calories	Fat Grams	Protein Grams	Carb Grams
MEAL #1: Stir egg whites together and pour into a lightly greased frying pan over medium heat. Add the cheese, bell pepper, tomatoes, and onions. Pull eggs toward the center until thoroughly cooked.					
Very lean protein	2 large egg whites	34	0.1	7.2	0.5
Medium-fat protein	1 oz 2% shredded cheese	80	6	7	0.5
Vegetable	3 tbs bell pepper	6	0.1	0.2	1.3
Vegetable	¼ cup tomato	7	0.1	0.3	1.5
Vegetable	1 oz white onion	10	0	0	2
Fruit	1 large (5.5 oz) peach	61	0.5	1.4	15.5
MEAL #2: Combine all ingredients for a salad.					
Vegetable	2 cups steamed bok choy	18	0.3	2.1	3.1
Starch	1 cup couscous	176	0.3	6	36.4
Vegetable	1 cup (6 oz) artichoke hearts	81	1	4.1	14.2
Vegetable	1 oz sun-dried tomatoes	73	0.9	4	15.8

Food		Calories	Fat Grams	Protein Grams	Carb Grams
MEAL #3: Stir-fry kale in oil with seeds before serving.					
Vegetable	2 cups chopped kale	67	0.9	4.4	13.4
Polyunsaturated	1 tbs sesame seeds	52	4.5	1.6	2.1
Polyunsaturated	1 tbs sesame seed oil	120	13.6	0	0
MEAL #4					
Very lean protein	4 oz roasted turkey breast	153	0.8	34	0
Vegetable	1 cup steamed broccoli	55	0.6	3.7	11.2
Medium-fat protein	2 pieces string cheese	120	5	14	1
MEAL #5					
Fruit	1 large (7.9 oz) apple	116	0.4	0.6	30.8
Vegetable	4.5 oz carrots	52	0.3	1.2	12.3
MEAL #6					
Very lean protein	4 oz lean top round, broiled	210	6.3	35.8	0
Vegetable	2 cups steamed turnip greens	58	0.6	3.3	12.7
Starch	6 oz baked or microwaved yam	197	0.2	2.5	46.9
Vegetable	1 cup steamed cauliflower	25	0.1	2	5.3
TOTAL		1832.6	42.6	135.4	226.5

DAY 4

Food		Calories	Fat Grams	Protein Grams	Carb Grams
MEAL #1: Combine ingredients in a single bowl.					
Low-fat milk	1 cup low-fat plain yogurt	154	3.9	12.9	17.2
Fruit	2.4 oz blueberries	39	0.2	2.5	9.9
Monounsaturated	1 oz almonds, raw unsalted	164	14.3	6	5.6
MEAL #2					
Fruit	1 (5.2 oz) nectarine	114	0.8	2.8	27.4
Very lean protein	1 oz nitrate-free turkey jerky	101.5	1	19.25	1

Food		Calories	Fat Grams	Protein Grams	Carb Grams
MEAL #3: Combine ingredients in a single bowl to create a salad.					
Vegetable	3 cups mixed green salad	20	0	1	3
Very lean protein	4 oz broiled chicken breast	186	4.1	35.1	0
Vegetable	½ cup tomato	16	0.2	0.8	3.5
Vegetable	½ cup cucumber	7	0.1	0.3	1.3
Free food	2 tbs fat-free Italian dressing	13	0.3	0.3	2.5
Vegetable	1 cup (1.5 oz)shredded red cabbage	13	0	0.5	3
Fruit	2.7 oz mandarin oranges	40	0.2	0.6	10.1
Soup/Starch	1.5 cups "Not So Portuguese" kale soup	102	2	3	18
MEAL #4					
Starch	1.5 cups cooked wild rice	248	0.7	9.8	52.4
Medium-fat protein	2 hard-boiled eggs	155	10.6	12.6	1.1
Fruit	1 cup strawberries	46	1	1	11.1
MEAL #5					
Very lean protein	4 oz mahi mahi, grilled	99	1	21.2	0
Vegetable	1 cup string beans	52	0.35	2.3	9.8
Vegetable	1 cup stewed tomatoes	80	2.7	2	13.2
Starch	2 slices Ezekiel bread	160	1	8	30
TOTAL		1848.7	44.45	141.95	220.1

Food		Calories	Fat Grams	Protein Grams	Carb Grams
MEAL #1					
Very lean protein	1 scoop whey protein drink	110	0.75	22	0.5
Monounsaturated	1 oz cashews, raw unsalted	157	12.4	8.6	5.2
Fruit	4 oz cherries	71	0.2	1.2	18.1
MEAL #2					
Vegetable	2 stalks celery	5	0.1	2	1.2
Monounsaturated	1 tbs natural reduced-fat peanut butter	100	6	4.5	6
Fruit	1 large (7.9 oz) apple	116	0.4	0.6	30.8
MEAL #3					
Starch	1 cup cooked brown basmati rice	216	2	5	45
Very lean protein	4 oz shrimp, grilled	112	1.2	23.7	0
Vegetable	8 asparagus spears, grilled	26	0.2	2.8	5
Vegetable	3 oz grilled eggplant	20	0.2	0.9	4.9
MEAL #4					
Very lean protein	¾ cup low-fat cottage cheese	153	3.2	23.3	6.1
Fruit	1cup/6oz peach	66	0.5	1.5	16.8
MEAL #5: Combine all ingredients to create a salad.					
Vegetable	2 cups shredded lettuce	32	0.6	6	2.4
Starchy vegetable	½ cup garbanzo beans	143	1.3	5.9	27.1
Vegetable	½ cup chopped tomato	16	0.2	0.8	3.5
Vegetable	½ cup cucumber	7	0.1	0.3	1.3
Vegetable	1 oz chopped red onion	12	0.1	0.3	2.9
Monounsaturated	2 oz olives	82	8.7	0.6	2.2
Polyunsaturated	2 tbs fat-free Italian dressing	13	0.3	0.3	2.5

Food		Calories	Fat Grams	Protein Grams	Carb Grams
MEAL #6					
Very lean protein	4 oz broiled halibut	158	3.3	30.3	0
Vegetable	1 cup/7.2 oz roasted butternut squash	82	0.2	1.8	21.5
Vegetable	1.5 cup kale, steamed	50	0.7	3.3	10
Vegetable	2 oz canned mushrooms, drained	14	0.2	1.1	2.9
TOTAL		1842.65	43.05	147.8	216.1

DAY 6

Food		Calories	Fat Grams	Protein Grams	Carb Grams
MEAL #1					
Lean Protein	3 oz smoked salmon	100	3.7	15.5	0
Saturated	1 tbs low-fat whippedcream cheese	23	1.8	1.1	0.7
Fruit	1 cup of grapes	104	0.3	1.1	27.3
Starch	2 slices whole-grain toast	113.5	1.5	5	20
MEAL #2					
Fruit	1 large (7.9 oz) apple	116	0.4	0.6	30.8
Monounsaturated	1 scoop whey protein drink	110	0.75	22	0.5
MEAL #3: Combine all ingredients to make a filling salad.					
Vegetables	3 cups mixed green salad	20	0	1	3
Very lean protein	1 can (3 oz) tuna in water	99	0.97	21.7	0
Starchy Vegetable	½ cup corn	66	0.9	2.5	14.6
Vegetable	2 tbs red pepper	5	0.1	0.2	1.1
Vegetable	1 oz chopped red onion	12	0.1	0.3	2.9
Vegetable	¼ cup cilantro	1	0.1	0.1	0.1
Vegetable	2 oz black beans	60	0.5	3.5	11.5
Monounsaturated	2 tbs oil and vinegar dressing	50	5	0	3

Food		Calories	Fat Grams	Protein Grams	Carb Grams
MEAL #4					
Lean protein	protein bar	240	7	18	26
Fruit	1 large (5.5 oz) peach	61	0.5	1.4	15.5
MEAL #5					
Lean protein	4 oz trout	192	8.2	27.5	0
Vegetable	2 cups cabbage	43	0.2	10	2.6
Vegetable	2 oz roasted red peppers	15	0.2	0.6	3.4
Starch	¼cup corn	33	0.5	1.2	7.3
Vegetable	¼ cup spinach	2	0.3	0.2	0.1
Starch	1 cup wild rice	166	0.5	6.5	34.9
MEAL #6					
Fruit	1 cup cherries	87	0.3	1.5	22.1
TOTAL		1695	33.8	139.5	227.4

Food		Calories	Fat Grams	Protein Grams	Carb Grams
MEAL #1					
Starch + very lean protein	Dr. Life'sprotein pancakes	351	6.5	32	42.1
Other sweet	¼ cup sugar-free syrup	35	0	0	12
MEAL #2					
Low-fat Milk	1 cup plain low fat yogurt	154	3.9	12.9	17.2
Fruit	½ cup blackberries	31	0.4	1	7.3
Monounsaturated	1 oz almonds, raw unsalted	164	14.3	6	5.6
MEAL #3					
Very lean protein	4 oz orange roughy, baked	119	1	25.6	0
Starch	6 oz yam	197	0.2	2.5	46.9
Vegetable	2 cups spinach	14	0.2	2.2	1.8
Vegetable	1 cup artichoke hearts	84	0.3	5.8	18.8

Food		Calories	Fat Grams	Protein Grams	Carb Grams
MEAL #4					
Medium fat protein	3 oz low-fat tofu	90	2	12	6
Fruit	1 medium (5.9 oz) pear	96	0.2	0.6	25.7
MEAL #5					
Very lean protein	4 oz very lean T-bone steak	200	8.4	29.4	0
Starch	¼ cup brown basmati rice	160	0	3	36
Vegetable	2 cups zucchini squash	40	0.5	3	8.4
Vegetable	1 cup brussels sprouts	56	0.8	4	11.1
TOTAL		1847.9	38.5	138.5	238.7

Diet based on 1800 Calories / 20% fat / 30% Protein / 50% Carbs

Feeling Hungry?

The Life Plan diets are meant to give you the right nutrients and enough calories to support your workouts and keep you feeling full all day long. But when you are training really hard, you might still be hungry, especially after you work out. The hunger you experience after workouts reflects the state of glycogen depletion you have created. This is exactly what you want. As you deplete your muscle and liver glycogen stores, your body is forced to use body fat for its energy, and this is what you need to lose body fat.

I view this hunger as a good thing. It tells me that I am burning fat and getting closer to my fat-loss goal. Once I began to think of hunger in a positive way, rather than as something I wanted to avoid, it became much easier to deal with.

However, you don't want to remain hungry for too long, because your body may begin breaking down muscle tissue instead of fat for energy. So, within one hour after an intense workout, you should have a protein/carb shake: 0.23 gram of protein and 0.7 gram of a high-glycemic-index carb per pound of body weight. In other words, if you're a 180-pound man, you should consume about 126 grams of carbs and 41 grams of protein. This will quickly replenish your glycogen stores, promote an anabolic hormonal environment for muscle building, and alleviate your hunger. And I would count this as one of your six meals for the day.

The Fat-Burning Diet

This fat-burning, low-glycemic option excludes red meat and dairy fat (such as cheese and milk). Just beyond the Basic Health Diet, this plan removes the biggest sources of saturated/plaque-building fat, which plugs your arteries. Eliminating this source will actually stop the progression of plaque—and in some cases, reverse plaque buildup.

While the commercial food industry is already doing a good job of removing trans fats from our food supply, no real effort is being made to rid our diets of saturated fats, which come almost exclusively from animal products. Other popular diets, such as Atkins and South Beach, center on low-glycemic carbohydrates, yet heart disease is still on the rise. To my mind, the combination of low-glycemic eating and consuming less than 10 percent of your calories from fat sets you on a heart-healthy path.

When I'm not extensively training, I follow this diet. When you are following the Fat-Burning Diet, you will be having five or six meals a day at three- to four-hour intervals. The recipes and menu suggestions for these healthy food choices can be easily prepared by steaming, grilling, or stir-frying with small amounts of oil. Follow this rotation for one week and then repeat. You can also mix up the days, but try to keep the meals together. At the end of the chapter, there are simple recipes that you can substitute if you prefer to cook your meals once a week, as I do.

FAT-BURNING DIET

Like the Basic Health Diet, many of these meals are self-explanatory and require no cooking and little preparation. Others require very rudimentary cooking skills, like chopping, baking, boiling, or broiling. Most of these meals can be prepared in a microwave oven. Just complete the instructions that precede the ingredients list to create a satisfying and easy-to-prepare single dish.

As in the previous diet, feel free to repeat days, but don't swap out individual meals.

DAY 1

Food		Calories	Fat Grams	Protein Grams	Carb Grams
MEAL #1: Combine the tofu, onions, and celery in a sauté pan over medium heat and cook. In a separate dish, prepare the oatmeal with the boiling water. Top with blueberries.					
Very lean protein	3 oz low-fat tofu	90	2	12	6
Vegetable	1 oz onion	12	0.1	0.3	2.9
Vegetable	1 oz celery	4	0.1	0.2	1
Fruit	5 oz blueberries	81	0.4	1	20.6

Food		Calories	Fat Grams	Protein Grams	Carb Grams
Starch	½ cup rolled oats	303	5.4	13.2	51.7
Free Food	1.5 cups boiling water				
MEAL #2					
Fruit	1 (5.2 oz) nectarine	114	0.8	2.8	27.4
Very lean protein	2 oz nitrate-free turkey jerky	203	2	38.5	2
MEAL #3					
Very lean protein	4 oz grilled tilapia	145	3.1	29.5	0
Soup/starch	1 cup lentil soup	150	2	9	28
Starch	¾ cup cooked brown rice	216	1.8	5	44.9
MEAL #4					
Very lean protein	1 scoop whey protein drink	110	0.75	22	0.5
Fruit	1 medium (6.4 oz) apple	95	0.4	0.5	25.1
MEAL #5: Combine all of these ingredients into one stir-fry.					
Very lean protein	5 oz shrimp	140	1.6	29.6	0
Vegetable	1.5 cup bok choy	14	0.2	1.6	2.3
Starchy vegetable	3 oz baby corn	45	0	8	3
Vegetable	1 cup snap peas	41	0.2	2.7	7.4
Vegetable	3 oz baby carrots	30	0.1	0.5	7
Free Food	2 tsp low-sodium soy sauce	6	0.1	0.5	0.9
TOTAL		1815.65	21.05	176.9	230.7

DAY 2

Food		Calories	Fat Grams	Protein Grams	Carb Grams
MEAL #1: Combine the Egg Beaters, tomato, onions, and cilantro in a sauté pan over medium heat and cook. In a separate dish, prepare the oatmeal with the soy milk. Top with blueberries.					
Very lean protein	½ cup Egg Beaters	60	0	12	2
Vegetable	½ cup tomato, diced	16	0.2	0.8	3.5
Vegetable	1 oz chopped red onion	12	0.1	0.3	2.9
Vegetable	cilantro (.1 oz)	1	0.1	0.1	0.1
Starch	¼ cup rolled oats	152	2.7	6.6	25.9

Food		Calories	Fat Grams	Protein Grams	Carb Grams
Fruit	1 oz blueberries	16	0.1	0.2	4.1
Medium-fat protein	½ cup soy milk	50	2	3.5	4
MEAL #2					
Very lean protein	1 scoop whey protein drink	110	0.75	22	0.5
Fruit	1.5 cups whole strawberries	69	0.6	1.4	16.6
MEAL #3: Combine all the ingredients exceptthe toast to create a filling salad.					
Very lean protein	4 oz grilled chicken breast	186	4.1	35.1	0
Vegetable	3 cups mixed green salad	20	0	1	3
Vegetable	½ cup tomato	16	0.2	0.8	3.5
Vegetable	½ cup cucumber	7	0.1	0.3	1.3
Vegetable	3 tbs bell pepper	6	0.1	0.2	1.3
Medium-fat protein	1 oz soy mozzarella	63	3	7	2
Vegetable	1 oz chopped red onion	12	0.1	0.3	2.9
Fruit	½ cup raspberries	32	0.4	0.7	7.3
Polyunsaturated	2 tbs raspberry vinaigrette	60	3	0	8
Starch	1 slice rye toast	160	0	6	34
MEAL #4					
Very lean protein	6 hard-boiled egg whites	102	0.6	21.6	1.2
Vegetable	1 oz white onion	10	0	0	2
Vegetable	¼ cup tomato	7	0.1	0.3	1.5
Vegetable	1 oz red peppers	7.5	0.1	0.3	1.7
Starch	1.5 cups cooked wild rice	248	0.7	9.8	52.4
MEAL #5					
Very lean protein	4 oz grilled mahi tuna	147	1.3	33.7	0
Starchy vegetable	1 sweet potato (6 oz)	162	0.4	3.6	37.3
Starch vegetable	1 cup snap peas	26	0.1	1.8	4.8
Vegetable	1 cup cauliflower	25	0.1	2	5.3
TOTAL		782.75	20.95	170.9	211.2

Food		Calories	Fat Grams	Protein Grams	Carb Grams
MEAL #1					
Very lean protein	2 scoops whey protein drink	220	1.5	44	1
Fruit	1 large (4.8 oz) banana	121	0.4	1.5	31
MEAL #2					
Monounsaturated	½ cup cubed avocado	120	11	1.5	6.4
Vegetable	¼ cup tomato	7	0.1	0.3	1.5
Vegetable	1 oz white onion	10	0	0	2
Very lean protein	1 oz nitrate-free turkey jerky	100	1	19	1
MEAL #3					
Very lean protein	4 oz broiled halibut	158	3.3	30.3	0
Vegetable	1 cup spinach	8	1.2	0.8	0.4
Starchy vegetable	7 oz yam, baked	230	0.2	3	54.8
Starchy vegetable	1 cup corn	66	1	2.4	14.6
MEAL #4					
Starchy vegetable	½ cup canned adzuki beans, rinsed and drained	147	0.1	8.6	28.5
Fruit	1 medium (4.6 oz) orange	62	0.1	1.2	15.5
MEAL #5					
Vegetable	1 can (11.5 oz) low-sodium V8 juice	72	0	2.9	14.4
Soup/starch	1.5 cups "Not So Portuguese" kale soup	102	2	3	18
MEAL #6					
Very lean protein	3.5 oz Alaskan crab	100	1.5	19	0
Vegetable	2 cups shredded bok choy	18	0.3	2.1	3.1
Starch	1 cup cooked couscous	176	0.3	6	36.4
Vegetable	1 cup (6 oz) artichoke hearts	84	0.3	5.8	18.8
TOTAL		1813.9	24.3	151.4	247.4

Food		Calories	Fat Grams	Protein Grams	Carb Grams
MEAL #1					
Very lean protein	4 large scrambled egg whites	69	0.3	14.4	0.9
Fruit	1 cup(8.1 oz) grapefruit sections	74	0.2	1.4	18.6
Fruit	1 cup (5.1 oz) blueberries	83	0.4	1.1	21
MEAL #2					
Lean protein	1 protein bar	240	7	18	26
Fruit	1 cup blackberries	62	0.7	2	14.7
MEAL #3					
Very lean protein	4 oz roasted turkey (white meat)	158	1.4	34.1	0
Vegetable	1 cup broccoli	55	0.6	3.7	11.2
Starchy vegetable	1.5 cups yellow squash	40	0	2	6
MEAL #4: Combine all ingredients for a filling snack					
Starchy vegetables	1 cup canned black beans, rinsed and drained	227	0.9	15.2	40.8
Vegetable	1 oz chopped red onion	12	0.1	0.3	2.9
Vegetable	½ cup tomato	16	0.2	0.8	3.5
MEAL #5					
Very lean protein	4 oz grilled chicken breast	186	4.1	35.1	0
Vegetable	1.5 cups boiled cabbage	50	0.9	2.3	10.1
Starch	1.5 cups cooked wild rice	248	0.7	0.7	52.4
Vegetable	1.5 cups cauliflower	38	0.2	3	8
MEAL #6					
Fruit	1 large apple (7.9 oz)	116	0.4	0.6	30.8
Very lean protein	1 scoop whey protein drink	110	0.75	22	0.5
TOTAL		1786.05	18.85	156.7	247.4

Food		Calories	Fat Grams	Protein Grams	Carb Grams

MEAL #1: Combine the oatmeal with the water and cook in a microwave oven on high for 3 minutes until the oatmeal absorbs the water to your preferred consistency. Top with sliced bananas. In a separate dish, prepare two hard-boiled eggs, eating only the whites.

Food		Calories	Fat Grams	Protein Grams	Carb Grams
Starch	½ cup dry old-fashioned oatmeal	152	2.7	6.6	25.9
Fruit	1 small (3.6 oz) banana	90	0.3	1.1	23
Very lean protein	6 egg whites	102	0.4	21.6	1.4
Free food	1.5 cups boiling water				
MEAL #2					
Vegetable	2 stalks celery	5	0.1	2	1.2
Monounsaturated	1 tbs natural reduced-fat peanut butter	100	6	4.5	6
Fruit	1 large (7.9 oz) apple	116	0.4	0.6	30.8

MEAL #3: Combine the shrimp with the vegetables to create a light salad.

Very lean protein	6 oz grilled shrimp	168	1.8	35.5	0
Vegetable	1 oz chopped red onion	12	0.1	0.3	2.9
Vegetable	2 tbs sweet relish	40	0.2	0.1	10.5
Starch	2 slices Ezekiel bread	160	1	8	30
Fruit	1 large (6.5 oz) orange	86	0.2	1.7	21.7
MEAL #4					
Fruit	1 cup blueberries	83	0.4	1.1	21
Fruit	1 cup strawberries	46	1	1	11.1
Monounsaturated	1 oz almonds	164	6	14.3	5.6
Very lean protein	1 oz nitrate-free turkey jerky	101.5	1	19.25	1

MEAL #5: Broil or grill the fish, zucchini, and eggplant for a few minutes on both sides until fully cooked.

Very lean protein	5 oz red snapper	142	1.8	29.1	0
Vegetable	4.4 oz zucchini	40	0.5	3	0.5
Vegetable	3 oz eggplant	20	0.2	0.9	4.9
Starchy vegetable	7 oz yam, baked or microwaved	230	0.2	3	54.8
TOTAL		184.6	24.3	153.15	254.5

Food		Calories	Fat Grams	Protein Grams	Carb Grams
MEAL #1: Combine egg whites, spinach, tomato, and onion in a heated sauté pan with the olive oil. Mix together until egg whites are fully cooked.					
Very lean protein	6 egg whites	102	0.4	21.6	1.4
Vegetable	1 cup spinach	7	0.1	0.9	1.1
Vegetable	¼ cup tomato	7	0.1	0.3	1.5
Vegetable	¼ cup onion	12	0.1	0.3	2.9
Monounsaturated	1 tsp olive oil	43	4.7	0	0
Fruit	1 medium (3.5 oz) fresh peach	38	0.3	0.9	9.7
MEAL #2					
Very lean protein	1 oz nitrate-free turkey jerky	100	1	18	1
Vegetable	1 cup (4.3 oz) carrots	50	0.8	1.1	11.7
Vegetable	1 cup cucumbers	14	0.2	0.7	2.6
MEAL #3: Combine all the ingredients for a filling salad.					
Very lean protein	½ cup cooked quinoa	127	2	4.5	23.5
Vegetable	2 oz roasted red peppers	15	0.2	0.6	3.4
Starch	¼ cup corn	33	0.5	1.2	7.3
Vegetable	¼ cup spinach	2	0.3	0.2	0.1
MEAL #4					
Very lean protein	4 oz turkey breast	153	0.8	34	0
Free food	1 tbs mustard	0	0	0	0
Starch	2 slices Ezekiel bread	160	1	8	30
Fruit	1 large (6.5 oz) orange	86	0.2	1.7	21.7
MEAL #5					
Soup/starch	1.5 cups "Not So Portuguese" kale soup	102	2	3	18
Very lean protein	3 oz seitan, warmed	150	1	18	3
Vegetable	1 cup string beans	34	1	2	7.8

Food		Calories	Fat Grams	Protein Grams	Carb Grams
MEAL #6					
Starch	1 cup cooked brown rice	216	1.8	5	44.9
Starchy vegetable	½ cup canned black beans, rinsed and drained	114	0.4	7.6	20.4
MEAL #7: Combine all the ingredients for a filling salad.					
Vegetable	3 cups mixed green salad	20	0	1	3
Very lean protein	4 oz grilled chicken breast	186	4.1	35.1	0
Vegetable	½ cup tomato	16	0.2	0.8	3.5
Vegetable	½ cup cucumber	7	0.1	0.3	1.3
Polyunsaturated	2 tbs fat-free Italian dressing	13	0.3	0.3	2.5
Vegetable	1 cup (1.5 oz) shredded red cabbage	13	0	0.5	3
Fruit	2.7 oz mandarin oranges	40	0.2	0.6	10.1
TOTAL		1828.6	23.8	168.2	235.4

DAY 7

Food		Calories	Fat Grams	Protein Grams	Carb Grams
MEAL #1: Combine the egg whites, peppers, tomato, and onions in a sauté pan over medium heat and cook. In a separate dish, prepare the oatmeal with the water to your desired consistency. Top with blueberries.					
Starch	¼ cup rolled oats	152	2.7	6.6	25.9
Fruit	2.4 oz blueberries	39	0.2	0.5	9.9
Very lean protein	5 egg whites	86	0.3	18	0
Vegetable	3 tbs bell pepper	6	0.1	0.2	1.3
Vegetable	¼ cup diced tomato	7	0.1	0.3	1.5
Vegetable	1 oz white onion	10	0	0	2
Free food	¾ cup boiling water				
MEAL #2					
Starchy vegetable	1 cup mung beans	160	0	0.3	19.5
Fruit	6 oz cherries	107	0.3	1.8	27.2
MEAL #3: Combine all ingredients for a delicious and filling salad.					
Very lean protein	4 oz tuna, canned	122	1.2	26.5	0
Vegetable	2 cups shredded lettuce	32	0.6	6	2.4

Food		Calories	Fat Grams	Protein Grams	Carb Grams
Starchy vegetable	½ cup garbanzo beans	143	1.3	5.9	27.1
Vegetable	½ cup chopped tomato	16	0.2	0.8	3.5
Vegetable	½ cup cucumber	7	0.1	0.3	1.3
Vegetable	1 oz chopped red onion	12	0.1	0.3	2.9
Polyunsaturated	2 tbs fat-free Italian dressing	13	0.3	0.3	2.5
MEAL #4					
Very lean protein	2 scoops whey protein drink	220	1.5	44	1
Monounsaturated	1 tbs natural reduced-fat peanut butter	100	6	4.5	6
Fruit	1 cup grapes	104	0.3	1.1	27.3
MEAL #5: Grill or broil the fish with the vegetables. Serve over rice.					
Very lean protein	4 oz haddock	127	1	27.5	0
Vegetable	1 cup brussels sprouts	56	0.8	4	11.1
Starchy vegetable	1.5 cups summer squash	30	0.4	2.3	6.3
Starch	1.25 cups cooked wild rice	207	0.6	8.2	43.7
TOTAL		1750.9	18.1	159.4	222.4

Heart Health Diet

This is my most extreme approach: a low-glycemic, vegetarian diet. The only good fats allowed are fish oil capsules. Poultry, fish, and nuts are allowed only if you cannot live without them, and then only in very small amounts.

This diet is definitely not for the first-time dieter, but it yields great results. This is a research-based plan that is perfect for men with known heart disease—those who have had angioplasty, stents, bypasses, or high coronary calcium scores. Significant research has shown that following this type of diet can reverse plaque and vascular disease.

The term "vegetarian" encompasses a wide range of dietary practices, including eating vegetables and no animal products (vegans), eating vegetables and dairy products with eggs (ovo-lacto vegetarians) or without eggs (lacto vegetarians), and eating vegetables with fish or poultry. A purely vegetarian approach (with less than 10 percent fat) is the only diet shown to reverse heart disease. Research in the last three years has demonstrated that vegetarians not only had more optimized cardiac function, but also improved vascular reactivity, lower blood pressure, balanced blood sugar levels, good cholesterol scores, and trimmer bodies.

If you are a vegan, the best way to make sure you get enough quality protein on this diet is to eat a variety of plant foods that have complementary amino acids. This can best be accomplished by eating a mixture of grains and legumes (rice and beans)—these contain all the essential amino acids that your body needs. Tofu is also an excellent source of high-quality plant protein because it contains all the essential amino acids and has a bonus of phytochemicals that protect you against heart disease and cancer. In addition, don't forget that nuts are an excellent source of protein, although they are high in fat. When you are following the Heart Health Diet, you will be having five or six meals a day at three- to four-hour intervals. The recipes and menu suggestions for these healthy food choices can be easily prepared by steaming, grilling, or stir-frying with small amounts of oil. At the end of the chapter, there are simple recipes that you can substitute if you prefer to cook your meals once a week, as I do.

HEART HEALTH DIET

DAY 1

Food		Calories	Fat Grams	Protein Grams	Carb Grams
MEAL 1: In a skillet, cook the tofu together with the onion and celery.					
Very lean protein	5 oz low-fat tofu	152	3.4	20.3	10.1
Vegetable	1 oz onion	12	0.1	0.3	2.9
Vegetable	1 oz celery	4	0.1	0.2	1
Fruit	5 oz blueberries	81	0.4	1	20.6
MEAL 2					
Vegetable	2 stalks celery	5	0.1	2	1.2
Vegetable	10 large baby carrots	53	0.2	1	12.3
Very lean protein	2 scoops whey protein drink	110	0.75	22	0.5
Fruit	1 large (7.4 oz) pear	121	0.8	0.8	32.4

Food		Calories	Fat Grams	Protein Grams	Carb Grams
MEAL 3					
High-fat starchy food	1 tbs hummus	50	3	1	5
Vegetable	3 oz baby carrots	30	0.1	0.5	7
Vegetable	1 cup sliced cucumbers	14	0.2	0.7	2.6
Starch	1 medium (2 oz) whole wheat pita	151	1.5	5.6	31.2
Fruit	1 cup grapes	104	0.3	1.1	27.3
MEAL 4: Combine these ingredients to make a hearty salad.					
Vegetable	3 cups mixed green salad	20	0	1	3
Vegetable	½ cup tomato	16	0.2	0.8	3.5
Vegetable	½ cup cucumber	7	0.1	0.3	1.3
Vegetable	3 tbs bell pepper	6	0.1	0.2	1.3
Lean protein	1 oz soy mozzarella	63	3	7	2
Vegetable	1 oz chopped red onion	12	0.1	0.3	2.9
Fruit	½ cup raspberries	32	0.4	0.7	7.3
Polyunsaturated	2 tbs raspberry vinaigrette	60	3	0	8
MEAL 5: Combine all ingredients as one stir-fry; heat in a pan until everything is fully cooked.					
Very lean protein	6 oz seitan	180	2	36	6
Vegetable	1.5 cups steamed bok choy	14	0.2	1.6	2.3
Starchy vegetable	3 oz baby corn	45	0	8	3
Vegetable	1 cup snap peas	41	0.2	2.7	7.4
Vegetable	3 oz baby carrots	30	0.1	0.5	7
	2 tsp low-sodium soy sauce	6	0.1	0.5	0.9
MEAL 6					
Very lean protein	2 scoops whey protein drink	220	1.5	44	1
Fruit	1 large (7.9 oz) apple	116	0.4	0.6	30.8
TOTAL		1811.15	22.35	160.7	241.8

Food		Calories	Fat Grams	Protein Grams	Carb Grams

MEAL 1: Combine the egg beaters, tomato, onions, and cilantro in a sauté pan over medium heat and cook. In a separate dish, prepare the oatmeal with the soy milk to your desired consistency. Top with blueberries.

Very lean protein	1 cup Egg Beaters	120	0	24	4
Vegetable	½ cup tomato	16	0.2	0.8	3.5
Vegetable	1 oz chopped red onion	12	0.1	0.3	2.9
Vegetable	¼ cup (.1 oz) cilantro	1	0.1	0.1	0.1
Starch	¼ cup rolled oats	152	2.7	6.6	25.9
Fruit	1 oz blueberries	16	0.1	0.2	4.1
Medium-fat protein	½ cup soy milk	50	2	3.5	4

MEAL 2

Lean protein	protein bar	240	7	18	26
Fruit	1.5 cups whole strawberries	69	0.6	1.4	16.6

MEAL 3: Sauté the tofu with the garlic and roasted red peppers until fully cooked.

Very lean protein	5 oz low-fat roasted tofu	152	3.4	20.3	10.1
Vegetable	1 tbs roasted garlic	13	0.1	0.5	2.8
Vegetable	1.5 oz roasted red pepper	11	0.1	0.4	2.6
Fruit	1 medium (6.4 oz) apple	95	0.4	0.5	25.1

MEAL 4

Soup/starch	1.5 cups "Not So Portuguese" kale soup	102	2	3	18
Starch	¾ cup cooked brown rice	162	1.3	3.8	33.6
Very lean protein	6 oz seitan, cooked	180	2	36	6

MEAL 5

Very lean protein	6 hard-boiled egg whites	102	0.6	21.6	1.2
Vegetable	1 oz white onion	10	0	0	2
Vegetable	¼ cup tomato	7	0.1	0.3	1.5
Vegetable	1 oz red peppers	7.5	0.1	0.3	1.7

MEAL 6: Combine all the ingredients in a sauté pan and cook until the kale has completely wilted.

Starchy vegetable	½ cup adzuki beans	147	0.2	8.6	28.5
Vegetable	1 tsp chopped garlic	4	0.1	0.2	0.9

Food		Calories	Fat Grams	Protein Grams	Carb Grams
Vegetable	1 tbs green onion	4	0.1	0.1	1
Vegetable	1 small (1.8 oz) grated carrot	21	0.1	0.5	4.8
Vegetable	1 tsp chopped ginger	2	0.1	0.1	0.4
Vegetable	1 cup steamed kale	34	0.5	2.2	6.7
TOTAL		1835	24	152.8	234

DAY 3

Food		Calories	Fat Grams	Protein Grams	Carb Grams
MEAL 1					
Very lean protein	2 scoops whey protein drink	220	1.5	44	1
Fruit	1 medium (4.2 oz) banana	105	0.4	1.3	26.9
MEAL 2					
Starch	1 medium (2 oz) whole wheat pita	151	1.5	5.6	31.2
Monounsaturated	½ avocado	161	14.8	2	8.5
Vegetable	¼ cup tomato	7	0.1	0.3	1.5
Vegetable	1 oz white onion	10	0	0	2
Very lean protein	6 oz seitan	180	2	36	6
MEAL 3: Combine these ingredients to create a filling salad.					
Vegetable	1 cup spinach	8	1.2	0.8	0.4
Starch	6 oz yam, baked or microwaved	197	0.2	2.5	46.9
Starchy vegetable	½ cup canned canelli beans, drained and rinsed	110	0	8	20
Vegetable	2 oz chopped onion	20	0	0	4
	1 tsp soy sauce	4	0.1	0.6	0.3
MEAL 4					
Very lean protein	4 hard-boiled egg whites	68	0.4	14.4	0.8
Vegetable	1 can (11.5 oz) low-sodium V8 juice	72	0	2.9	14.4

Food		Calories	Fat Grams	Protein Grams	Carb Grams
MEAL 5: Combine all of these ingredients for a filling salad.					
Vegetable	2 cups shredded bok choy	18	0.3	2.1	3.1
Starch	1 cup cooked couscous	176	0.3	6	36.4
Vegetable	1 cup (6 oz) artichoke hearts	81	1	4.1	14.2
Vegetable	1 oz sun-dried tomatoes	73	0.9	4	15.8
Starchy vegetable	½ cup adzuki beans	147	0.2	8.6	28.5
TOTAL		1844.5	24.9	143.2	261.9

DAY 4

Food		Calories	Fat Grams	Protein Grams	Carb Grams
MEAL 1: Combine the oats and water and cook until your desired consistency is reached. Top with blueberries. In a lightly greased separate pan, scramble the egg whites.					
Starch	¼ cup rolled oats	152	2.7	6.6	25.9
Very lean protein	3 egg whites	51	0.2	10.8	0.7
Fruit	1 cup blueberries	83	0.4	1.1	21
Free food	¾ cup boiling water				
MEAL 2					
Vegetable	2 stalks celery	5	0.1	2	1.2
Monounsaturated	2 tbs natural reduced-fat peanut butter	200	12	9	12
Very lean protein	2 scoops whey protein drink	220	1.5	44	1
MEAL 3					
Soup/starch	1.5 cups "Not So Portuguese" kale soup	102	2	3	18
Very lean meat	3 oz seitan	150	1	18	3
Fruit	1 small peach	31	0.2	0.7	7.8
MEAL 4: Combine these ingredients in a large sauté pan and cook until the kale is wilted.					
Starchy vegetable	1 cup canned black beans, rinsed and drained	227	0.9	15.2	40.8
Vegetable	1 oz chopped red onion	12	0.1	0.3	2.9
Vegetable	½ cup tomato	16	0.2	0.8	3.5
Vegetable	2 cups collard greens	25	0	2	5

Food		Calories	Fat Grams	Protein Grams	Carb Grams
MEAL 5					
Vegetable	1.5 cups boiled cabbage	50	0.9	2.3	10.1
Starch	1.25 cups cooked wild rice	207	0.6	8.2	43.7
Vegetable	1.5 cups cauliflower	38	0.2	3	8
MEAL 6: Combine all ingredients for a hearty salad.					
Vegetable	3 cups chopped watercress	11	0.1	2.3	1.3
Fruit	1 oz dried apricot	67	0.1	0.9	17.5
Vegetable	½ cup chopped tomato	16	0.2	0.8	3.5
Vegetable	½ cup cucumber	7	0.1	0.3	1.3
Vegetable	1 oz chopped red onion	12	0.1	0.3	2.9
Very lean protein	4 hard-boiled egg whites	68	0.4	14.2	0.8
TOTAL		1796.6	25	145.8	231.9

DAY 5

Food		Calories	Fat Grams	Protein Grams	Carb Grams
MEAL 1: Combine the oatmeal and water in a microwave-safe dish, and heat on high for 3 minutes or until the desired consistency is reached. Top with sliced bananas. In a separate pan, hard-boil the egg, but eat only the whites.					
Starch	½ cup dry old-fashioned oatmeal	152	2.7	6.6	25.9
Fruit	1 small (3.6 oz) banana	90	0.3	1.1	23
Very lean protein	6 egg whites	102	0.4	21.6	1.4
Free food	1.5 cups water				
MEAL 2					
Vegetable	2 stalks celery	5	0.1	2	1.2
Fruit	1 medium (6.4 oz) apple	95	0.4	0.5	25.1
Very lean protein	2 scoops whey protein drink	220	1.5	44	1
MEAL 3					
Starch	1 cup cooked brown rice	216	1.8	5	44.9
Starchy vegetable	½ cup canned black beans, drained and rinsed	114	0.4	7.6	20.4

Food		Calories	Fat Grams	Protein Grams	Carb Grams
MEAL 4					
Vegetable	1 oz chopped red onion	12	0.1	0.3	2.9
Vegetable	2 tbs sweet relish	40	0.2	0.1	10.5
Vegetable	2 oz sliced cucumber	7	0.1	0.3	1.2
Vegetable	1 oz sliced tomato	5	0.1	0.3	1.2
Starchy vegetable	½ oz bean sprouts	9	0.1	0.9	1.7
Starch	2 slices Ezekiel bread	160	1	8	30
Starchy vegetable	½ cup edamame	127	5.8	11.1	10
MEAL 5					
Very lean protein	1 scoop whey protein drink	110	0.75	22	0.5
MEAL 6					
Vegetable	4.3 oz grilled portobello mushroom	42	1	4.9	1
Vegetable	4.1 oz grilled asparagus	26	2.9	2.9	4.9
Vegetable	4.4 oz grilled zucchini	40	0.5	3	0.5
Vegetable	3 oz grilled eggplant	20	0.2	0.9	4.9
Starch	6 oz baked yam	197	0.2	2.5	46.9
TOTAL		1806.45	20.55	145.6	241.2

DAY 6

Food		Calories	Fat Grams	Protein Grams	Carb Grams
MEAL 1: In a heated skillet, heat the olive oil and then add in the egg whites, spinach, tomato, and onion and cook thoroughly.					
Very lean protein	6 egg whites	102	0.4	21.6	1.4
Vegetable	1 cup spinach	7	0.1	0.9	1.1
Vegetable	¼ cup tomato	7	0.1	0.3	1.5
Vegetable	¼ cup onion	12	0.1	0.3	2.9
Fruit	1 medium (3.5 oz) fresh peach	38	0.3	0.9	9.7
	Olive oil				

Food		Calories	Fat Grams	Protein Grams	Carb Grams
MEAL 2					
Very lean protein	2 scoops whey protein drink	220	1.5	44	1
Vegetable	carrots (4.3 oz)	50	0.8	1.1	11.7
Vegetable	cauliflower (3.5 oz)	25	0.1	2	5.3
Polyunsaturated	2 tbs low-fat ranch dressing for dipping	80	7	1	3
MEAL 3: Combine all the ingredients in a stockpot to make a soup. Cook over high heat until broth boils.					
Vegetable	1 cup boiled kale	19	0.6	1	3.3
Vegetable	1 tbs white onion	4	0.1	0.1	1
Soup/starch	1 cup vegetable broth	15	0	0	3
Starchy vegetables	½ cup cannellini beans	110	0	8	20
Vegetable	½ cup sliced carrots	26	0.1	0.6	6.1
MEAL 4: Combine the beans, garlic, green onions, carrots, kale, and ginger in a sauté pan and cook until the kale has wilted.					
Starchy vegetable	½ cup adzuki beans, drained and rinsed	147	0.1	8.6	28.5
Vegetable	1 tsp chopped garlic	4	0.1	0.2	0.9
Vegetable	1 tbs green onion	4	0.1	0.1	1
Vegetable	1 small (1.8 oz) grated carrot	21	0.1	0.5	4.8
Vegetable	1 tsp chopped ginger	2	0.1	0.1	0.4
Starchy	1 cup cooked wild rice	166	0.5	6.5	34
Vegetable	1 cup kale	34	0.5	2.2	6.7
MEAL 5					
Vegetable	2 cups shredded bok choy	18	0.3	2.1	3.1
Vegetable	1 cup (6 oz) artichoke hearts	81	1	4.1	14.2
Vegetable	1 oz sun-dried tomatoes	73	0.9	4	15.8
MEAL 6					
Starchy vegetable	1 cup baked butternut squash	82	0.2	1.8	21.5
Vegetable	8 grilled asparagus spears (2.1 oz)	26	0.2	2.9	4.9

Food		Calories	Fat Grams	Protein Grams	Carb Grams
Starchy vegetable	¾ cup white beans, drained and rinsed	187	0.5	13.1	33.7

MEAL 7: Combine all ingredients for a filling salad.

Vegetable	3 cups mixed green salad	20	0	1	3
Vegetable	½ cup tomato	16	0.2	0.8	3.5
Vegetable	½ cup cucumber	7	0.1	0.3	1.3
Polyunsaturated	2 tbs fat-free Italian dressing	13	0.3	0.3	2.5
Vegetable	1 cup (1.5 oz)shredded red cabbage	13	0	0.5	3
Very lean protein	4 egg whites	68.5	0	14.4	0
TOTAL		1786.3	21.1	145.3	253.8

DAY 7

Food		Calories	Fat Grams	Protein Grams	Carb Grams

MEAL 1: Combine oatmeal and water in a microwave-safe dish and cook on high for 3 minutes or until the desired consistency is met. Top with blueberries. In a separate pan, scramble the egg whites and remaining ingredients.

Starch	¼ cup rolled oats	152	2.9	6.6	25.9
Free food	¾ cup water				
Fruit	2.4 oz blueberries	39	0.2	0.5	9.9
Very lean protein	5 egg whites	86	0.3	18	0
Vegetable	3 tbs bell pepper	6	0.1	0.2	1.3
Vegetable	¼ cup diced tomato	7	0.1	0.3	1.5
Vegetable	1 oz white onion	10	0	0	2

MEAL 2

Very lean protein	2 scoops whey protein drink	220	1.5	44	1
Fruit	6 oz cherries	107	0.3	1.8	27.2

MEAL 3: Combine all the ingredients for a filling salad.

Vegetable	2 cups shredded lettuce	32	0.6	6	2.4
Starchy vegetable	½ cup garbanzo beans	143	1.3	5.9	27.1
Vegetable	½ cup chopped tomato	16	0.2	0.8	3.5

Food		Calories	Fat Grams	Protein Grams	Carb Grams
Vegetable	½ cup cucumber	7	0.1	0.3	1.3
Vegetable	1 oz chopped red onion	12	0.1	0.3	2.9
Polyunsaturated	2 tbs fat-free Italian dressing	13	0.3	0.3	2.5
MEAL 4					
Very lean protein	2 scoops whey protein drink	220	1.5	44	1
Monounsaturated	1 tbs natural reduced-fat peanut butter	100	6	4.5	6
Fruit	1 cup grapes	104	0.3	1.1	27.3
MEAL 5: Combine all the vegetables in a sauté pan and cook until softened. Serve over the rice.					
Starchy vegetable	1 cup black-eyed peas, drained and rinsed	180	2	12	32
Vegetable	1 oz chopped yellow onion	12	0.1	0.3	2.9
Vegetable	2 oz green pepper	11	0.1	0.5	2.6
Starchy vegetable	½ cup summer squash	30	0.4	2.3	6.3
Starch	1.25 cups cooked wild rice	207	0.6	8.2	43.7
TOTAL		1795.8	18.8	157.9	230.3

No dairy, no meat, no poultry, no fish, or egg yolks

Diet based on 1800 Calories / 10% fat / 35% Protein / 55% Carbs

Become a Bag Man

We all know that protein is essential for building and maintaining muscle mass, but most of us find it difficult to get optimal protein when we're rushing about during the day. It's time to rethink that. Healthy eating is possible—no matter how busy you are.

My wife, Annie, has made dieting effortless for me. She has come up with her own creation, and it has revolutionized my ability to stay on track with my nutrition program. If you start following her lead, you will never find yourself without healthy food.

First, you'll need a food vacuum sealer. It is very simple to operate and will save you time and money because you buy food in large quantities. Annie prepares my "protein packs" once a week. It saves her an enormous amount of cooking/prep time and yields about 21 (6-ounce) servings of protein. I keep some at home and take several to work with me and keep them frozen until ready to use. To cook, I simply make a small cut in the bag, just enough to release steam. I then microwave for 2 to 3 minutes, depending on the thickness of the fish. Then I let it stand for 1 minute in the bag before serving. It can be served on a bed of thinly sliced Napa cabbage or brown rice. This same process can be used for cooked brown/wild rice.

I also have several frozen individual servings of vegetables I get at the grocery store, which can quickly be prepared, creating a completely balanced meal: 1 bag of protein, 1 bag of low-glycemic carb (yam, wild rice, or brown rice), and a serving of healthy vegetables.

SALT—HOW MUCH IS TOO MUCH?

Most of us really don't have to worry about how much salt we eat. About 20 percent of our population is salt-sensitive, and when these people consume salt they retain excess fluid. This extra fluid leads to an increase in their circulatory volume, which, in turn, increases the work their hearts must perform and can also increase their blood pressure.

If you are not salt-sensitive and don't have a family history of hypertension (high blood pressure), I think you can continue to use salt in cooking and buy foods that have sodium in them as long as you do so in moderation. However, you need to recognize that most men eat way too much salt. I have found that if you do cut down on salt you will begin to appreciate other flavors in foods a lot more and become less inclined to crave processed foods or fast foods.

The Life Plan Recipes

Almost all of these very simple recipes can be used on any of the diets. The following notations indicate the diet plan that applies to each: Basic Health Diet (BHD), Fat-Burning Diet (FBD), and Heart Health Diet (HHD). Unless otherwise noted, all recipes are for single servings, and can be doubled or tripled if you want to prepare your food ahead, or if you are entertaining a friend.

Breakfast Options

EGG WHITE OMELET WITH FRESH HERBS (BHD, FBD, HHD)

4 egg whites with 2 tbs water

1 cup chopped fresh spinach leaves

½ bunch fresh parsley (½ cup)

1 tbs fresh basil, chopped

4 tsp chopped green onion

2 tsp chopped chives

1 tbs fresh chopped dill

Combine all herbs and spinach in bowl, then mix. Beat egg whites and water until fluffy. Spray skillet with nonstick cooking spray and heat over medium-low heat. Add herb mixture to egg whites and very lightly stir. Pour mixture into skillet and cover. Cook slowly until the egg is almost set. With rubber spatula, fold omelet in half and cook an additional minute. Serve immediately.

MY FAVORITE BREAKFAST (BHD, FBD, HHD)

4 ice cubes in the blender

½ cup of nonfat half-&-half

⅔ cup cold coffee

1½ scoops of Chocolate Protein Powder

1 6-inch banana

Blend for 1 to 2 minutes. This is typically my first meal of the day and I drink it after my resistance training session.

DR. LIFE'S PANCAKE (BHD, FBD, HHD)

½ cup natural oatmeal

1 cup egg whites

1 tbs sugar-free maple syrup

Mix ingredients in blender, then fry in pan with nonfat spray.

"NOT SO PORTUGUESE" KALE SOUP (BHD, FBD, HHD)

One of my favorite New England dishes is Portuguese kale soup—but it's high in fat. Try my tasty, healthier version. This recipe will make a large batch that will last for several days if refrigerated, and longer if frozen.

2 large (48 oz) cans of 100% fat-free, low-sodium beef or vegetable broth

1 large yellow onion (chopped)

4–6 cloves fresh garlic, minced

1½ tsp crushed red pepper

2 cans cannellini beans (rinsed/drained)

1–2 lb fresh kale (stems removed/cut)

Black pepper and/or paprika to taste

In a large soup kettle, sauté onions in ¼ cup of the broth. Add the remaining broth, red pepper, and garlic. Add the beans and kale, bring to a boil, then stir and lower the heat. Cook just long enough until the kale is tender, about 3 to 4 minutes.

GRILLED SQUASH WITH ASPARAGUS (BHD, FBD, HHD)

1 large zucchini (washed/cut in ¼-inch diagonal slices)

1 large yellow summer squash (washed/cut in ¼-inch diagonal slices)

1 lb fresh asparagus (diagonally cut into 2-inch pieces)

1 bunch fresh basil

Medium red onion (thinly sliced)

Crushed red pepper flakes

Warm grill to medium heat. Mix veggies together and sprinkle with crushed red pepper flakes to taste. You can use just a spritz of extra virgin olive oil or spray. Add fresh basil leaves (whole). Place all ingredients in a nonstick grill wok and grill 15 to 20 minutes, stirring often until tender.

LEMON/DILL CHICKEN BREAST (BHD, FBD, HHD)

This recipe can be doubled or tripled and individually portioned and frozen after cooking.

4 (6 oz) chicken breasts (boneless/skinless)

1 lemon (cut in half)

1 teaspoon paprika

8 small sprigs of fresh dill

4 tbs capers, rinsed (to reduce sodium)

Rinse and tenderize chicken breasts. Sprinkle with paprika and squeeze juice from ½ lemon over breasts. Place breasts on aluminum foil. Broil 6 to 8 minutes or until lightly browned. Flip breasts and broil an additional 6 to 8 minutes until lightly browned. Remove from broiler. On each breast, place a few sprigs of fresh dill weed. Next, place 2 or 3 very thin slices of lemon on top of the dill, and 1 tablespoon of capers on top of that. Return to broiler and broil an additional 1 to 2 minutes.

Dinner Options

QUICK SESAME GINGER SALMON (BHD, FBD, HHD)

4 lb of wild Alaskan salmon cut into 6 oz portions (approx. 10 servings)

½ tsp of Iron Chef Brand Sesame Garlic Sauce* spread over each piece

1 tsp Eden Shake seasoning* sprinkled on each piece

Place 1 raw seasoned salmon in each bag and vacuum seal according to directions. Freeze. To prepare the individual serving, simply remove from freezer 15 minutes before cooking. Oven: Broil on high or microwave until fish flakes. Make a small cut in the corner of the bag to release pressure and microwave on high for 2 minutes, then flip and microwave 2 more minutes. (Microwave oven temperatures may vary and can require an extra minute on each side.)

Readily available in the international section of most grocery or natural food stores.

BAKED STUFFED WILD SALMON FILLET (BHD, FBD, HHD)

This recipe can be doubled or tripled and individually portioned and frozen after cooking.

6 fresh wild salmon fillets (6 oz each)

4–6 cups fresh baby spinach

4 cloves garlic (thinly sliced)

½ cup slivered water chestnuts

1 cup thinly sliced white mushrooms

Olive oil cooking spray

Fresh ground pepper

Preheat oven to 400 degrees. Mix spinach, water chestnuts, garlic, and mushrooms together in bowl. Very lightly spray baking dish or cookie sheet with olive oil spray. Place salmon fillets on prepared dish. Divide spinach mixture evenly on each fillet and roll. Be sure to place seam side down. Top each roll with freshly ground pepper as desired. Bake 8–10 minutes or until fish flakes easily when fork is inserted.

STEAMED TILAPIA FILLETS (BHD, FBD, HHD)

This recipe can be doubled or tripled and individually portioned and frozen after cooking.

1 (6 oz) tilapia fillet

1 tsp fat-free mayonnaise

Juice from fresh lemon

2 sprigs of fresh dill per fillet

Fresh ground pepper to taste

Put approximately 3 inches of water in bottom of steamer pot. Place fillets in top steamer pan. With a pastry brush, spread mayonnaise over fillets. Squeeze lemon juice over each, garnishing with sprigs of fresh dill. Grind fresh pepper to taste.

Place lid on pan and heat on high until water boils and heavy steam begins. Turn heat to medium and steam for 20 minutes or until fish flakes easily.

CHOCOLATE BANANA PROTEIN SHAKE (BHD, FBD, HHD)

1–2 scoops (chocolate) Life Plan Shake 8 oz water 4 ice cubes 1 banana	Blend on high speed for about 30 seconds.

SLICED APPLE WITH NATURAL PEANUT BUTTER (BHD, FBD)

1 medium apple 1 tbs natural peanut butter	Wash and slice apple. Spread each apple slice with a little bit of the peanut butter and enjoy. Natural peanut butter has no added sugar or salt. Its only ingredient is ground peanuts. It is available at all natural food stores and many grocery stores. Be sure to keep it refrigerated between uses.

The Life Plan Is Forever

I have learned over the years from my patients and my own experiences that once most of us reach our fat-loss/muscle-building goals we celebrate by returning to our old habits. It's truly amazing how little time it takes before we can look just like our "before" photos. That's why all three of the diets you've read about are "forever." There is no such thing as a maintenance program on the Life Plan.

If you are anything like me, you will periodically get off track. Make sure that you recognize this right away, and get your act together and get back on the diet as soon as possible. Don't wait for "the end of the week" or the start of business on Monday: You don't have this luxury. The more time you spend off track, the harder it will be to get back on.

Once you have reached your goals, continue to monitor your body fat percentage, muscle mass, strength, and all of your biomarkers for disease at least every three months. Get new bathing suit photos of yourself every three months and post them right next to your "before" photo on your refrigerator door, or in your wallet. You don't want to ever forget how you used to look and feel. If you follow these suggestions, I think you will stay on the right track to a lifetime of leanness, great appearance, and good health.

THE LIFE PLAN
WORKOUTS

CHAPTER 4

The Importance of Exercise

- -

My workouts take me to a unique mental zone where my life is redefined and given rhythm, order, balance, and flow. Yet it didn't start out that way. It's hard to believe when you look at me now, but not so many years ago it was more than a struggle to get myself out of bed and into the gym. I had to constantly create goals and incentives to keep me going. But after a while, I was reveling in the joy of my success: I just had to look in the mirror to see what I had accomplished. More than that, for the first time in my life, I felt great physically and emotionally. And I knew that my good health was mostly due to my exercise routine.

That's why exercise is the cornerstone of my Life Plan: Without it, there is no way that I could continue to look and feel like I do at age 72. Even if you replace diminishing hormones and follow healthy eating habits, you can't experience active aging without exercising every day. You need the right regimen and the right intensity to succeed. Once you start feeling younger and looking better, you won't ever want to stop. This is especially true because exercise is better than anything else you can do to enhance your sex life.

Exercise and Sexual Function
- -

Having sex three times a week serves as a benchmark that you're healthy and physically fit. If you're not keeping up, you may be out of shape in more ways than you thought. Sex is a form of physical exertion that can be harmful to men with advanced heart disease, especially if you're not in shape. A study of healthy married men (ages 25 to 43) showed that the highest recorded heart rate during sex was 127 beats per minute—that's 67 percent of maximum heart rate, which is a high rate for the nonathletic.

The strength of your erection is a true barometer of your overall health. But here's the problem: An estimated 34 percent of all American men age 40 to 70 suffer from some level of erectile dysfunction. Before you fill your Viagra prescription, or talk to your doctor about getting one, there's plenty you can do yourself to get your sex life back on track.

The latest research suggests that exercise helps improve male sexual function. According to the chief exercise physiologist for the American Council on Exercise, Dr. Cedric Bryant, improving muscle strength and tone, endurance, body composition, and cardiovascular function is key to a prolonged sex life. Physically active men over 50 reported better erections—and had a 30 percent lower risk for impotence than their inactive cohorts. Other research studied over 40,000 men and became the largest study to demonstrate that the more exercise a man does, the less likely he'll experience erectile dysfunction. Plus, exercise boosts you psychologically, reducing stress, increasing confidence, and elevating moods.

Every aspect of the Life Plan will improve your sex life. Here's how your sexual health will benefit from following my program:

Flexibility/balance: Flexibility is one of the most important components of sexual fitness—and one of the most ignored. Exercise that mimics everyday life is what you need to focus on to improve your sexual function. For example, bending over to pick something off the floor, reaching, swinging, pushing, and pulling all increase your flexibility. These are called functional workouts, which you will learn more about in Chapter 5. They train your body to move in all planes of motion: forward, backward, rotation, and lateral.

Resistance training: Lifting heavy weights and performing compound movements (squats, dead lifts, and bench presses) increases serum testosterone and growth hormone levels—key hormones to improve sexual function.

Cardio: Working out at an intensity level of 65 to 85 percent of maximum heart rate (which I discuss in Chapter 7) can mean no ED problems, according to a nine-year study published in the August 2000 issue of *Urology* by Dr. Irwin Goldstein, Boston University School of Medicine. Investigators also found that men who continued or started working out as late as middle age were still able to lower their impotence risk.

Exercise Actively Combats Disease

Good health is far more than an active sex life and the absence of disease—it's the ability to maintain strength, movement, and balance. Once you master these three components, you'll be able to continue living your life to the fullest and avoid getting old. Exercise is the vehicle that gets you there and keeps you there.

In reality, physical exercise is just another medical protocol. A 2002 study published in the *New England Journal of Medicine* concluded that exercise capacity is perhaps the most powerful predictor of life span. Exercise has also proven to be an effective strategy for preventing or reversing the top killers of American men:

- **Arthritis:** Men with rheumatoid or degenerative arthritis benefit from exercise, which improves endurance, strengthens muscles, and increases both joint flexibility and range of motion. These benefits can't be realized with drugs or surgery.

- **Cancer:** Evidence suggests physical activity reduces the risk for colon cancer.

- **Cerebrovascular disease:** Exercise restores function following a stroke—a benefit not shared by drugs or surgery.

- **Chronic obstructive pulmonary disease (COPD):** Adding exercise to a COPD rehabilitation program can result in both physiological and psychological benefits, even for those with severe air flow obstruction or asthma.

- **Coronary artery disease:** Exercise combined with the right nutritional therapy can reverse heart disease, the number-one killer of all Americans. It also improves heart function, reduces several coronary risk factors, enhances psychosocial well-being after a heart attack, and improves long-term survival. Both resistance training and cardiovascular workouts strengthen the heart muscle.

- **Depression:** Aerobic exercises like walking and running reduce depression and anxiety, improve stress tolerance, enhance self-image, and increase one's sense of well-being. Plus, exercise stimulates the release of your own "feel-good" hormones (endorphins).

- **Diabetes:** Exercise can prevent, delay, or even reverse the serious complications of diabetes, namely, vascular disease of the brain, heart, kidneys, eyes, and legs.

- **Dyslipidemia:** Abnormalities of blood fats (high total cholesterol, LDL, and triglycerides and low HDL cholesterol) are major risk factors for vascular disease of the heart, brain, kidneys, eyes, and legs. Regular exercise reduces total cholesterol and triglyceride levels, raises HDL cholesterol, and lowers LDL.

- **Hypertension:** Aerobic exercise and resistance training can help reduce blood pressure. Many men who adhere to a regular, specifically prescribed aerobic exercise program like mine can reduce their blood pressure without taking drugs—avoiding potentially toxic side effects and the considerable expense of long-term drug therapy.

- **Obesity:** Daily exercise is an essential strategy for achieving and maintaining optimal weight.

- **Osteoporosis:** High-intensity strength training will prevent and actually reverse bone loss and other degenerative bone diseases.

- **Sarcopenia:** Resistance training prevents muscle loss that accompanies aging, a major cause of disability and premature death.

Nate Exercised His Way out of Bone Loss

Nate, a 58-year-old patient, was shocked to discover he had osteoporosis in his hips and lumbar spine. A thin guy, at 5-11 and 170 pounds, Nate never thought he had health issues. But his slim build and low testosterone levels fit the profile of the typical man with early onset osteoporosis. I told Nate that the best way for him to reverse bone loss was to start a vigorous resistance training program. I also started him on hormone therapy to replace his testosterone and thyroid hormone deficiencies, and I had him follow my Life Plan Diet. Within one year, he was able to reverse his osteoporosis.

Sarcopenia: Every Man's Dilemma

As we age, the most dramatic and significant decline we experience is in our lean body mass and strength. These two muscular functions ultimately determine our quality of life. And nowhere is this more evident than in the aging syndrome known as sarcopenia, the loss of muscle mass.

Sarcopenia is defined as having an 18 percent or greater loss of lean body mass when compared to men in their 20s. It accounts for decreases in basal metabolic rate (BMR), muscle strength, and overall activity levels. As your BMR declines, so do your energy requirements. However, most men don't reduce caloric intake as they age, causing body fat to gradually increase each year as they lose muscle tissue. For example, the average 25-year-old man has 20 percent body fat, but by 55 that jumps to 30 percent and by 75 it's 35 percent. It typically begins in your early 40s, progressing at 3 to 5 percent for that decade and increasing to 10 or 20 percent per decade after 50. The average man can expect to gain roughly one pound of fat every year between the ages of 30 and 60, while losing about a half pound of muscle mass each year.

The problem with this equation is that it affects not only the way you look, but the way you feel and how fast you age. The pounds you gain are making you look older and out of shape, and affect every other aspect of your health. At the same time, the loss of muscle mass makes you look and feel weak because

THE LINK BETWEEN INSULIN, HEART DISEASE, AND EXERCISE

Elevated fasting insulin level (hyperinsulinemia) may be the most powerful predictor of heart disease. Constant surges of blood sugar ensue, rendering insulin less able to do its job and requiring more of it to meet our daily metabolic needs. This vicious cycle slowly cripples the immune system, makes you fat, increases your blood pressure, and brings on serious degenerative diseases, including the major cause of death in this country—heart disease.

Both aerobic and resistance training can help reverse insulin resistance. The more you burn fat (as opposed to glycogen) for energy during aerobic training, the more sensitive you become to the insulin your body produces. As your body fat disappears and your muscle mass increases, your insulin resistance diminishes, taking a huge burden off your pancreas so it can now secrete less insulin throughout the day. The greater your sensitivity to insulin, the more effective you become at removing sugar from your blood, keeping blood sugars and insulin levels in a healthy range and burning your own body fat for energy.

you *are* getting weaker. From age 60 onward, your energy levels will decline and frailty ensues, affecting your bones and your ability to move around. The largest loss of muscle mass occurs between the ages of 50 and 75—with an average loss of 25 percent. Mostly the disease involves type II (fast-twitch) muscle fibers, which are linked to strength.

What Causes Sarcopenia?

Generally speaking, six areas contribute to the disease:

- Diminished protein metabolism

- Decline in natural hormone levels

- Spinal cord changes

- Decline in physical activity

- Poor nutrition

- Cellular dysfunction

Sarcopenia and Cellular Dysfunction

The mitochondria, the powerhouses of the cell, are the principal sites where your energy, in the form of adenosine 5'-triphosphate or ATP, is generated. Free radicals, the unstable atoms that react with other compounds, are produced primarily in the mitochondria when the food you eat is converted to energy. These atoms attack other molecules in order to gain stability and damage and destroy mitochondria in the process. Mitochondrial damage leads to impaired ATP production, cellular breakdown, and sarcopenia, among other diseases, as well as early aging.

Gene Shifting

The good news is that you don't have to accept weakness and frailty as the status quo of aging. Instead, I'll show you how to replace your old, worn-out, damaged, and dying mitochondria with brand-new, wild-type mitochondria (the scientific name for young mitochondria) and regain your muscle mass and strength. It's all done through a process called gene shifting, which transforms our damaged, mutated, dying mitochondria into young, healthy wild-type mitochondria to prevent or even reverse sarcopenia.

It all starts with exercise—specifically heavy resistance exercise. You'll learn exactly how to do this in Chapter 6, where you will be working with fairly heavy weights and train to muscle failure. This type of exercise can offer you the best opportunity to experience a transformation in your mitochondria: Intense resistance training induces adaptations in our mitochondria that can reverse the progression of aging. Some recent studies have actually shown that with just two months of strength training, men can reverse two decades of muscle loss. Other studies have shown resistance training can significantly increase our type II fiber cross-sectional area and increase mitochondrial volume in older adults.

Once you have incorporated resistance training into your exercise routine, you will have increased strength, which then improves daily living and overall quality of life and keeps you from getting old. You can experience this change just as easily as many of my patients. For example, Frank, a 77-year-old patient, followed the Life Plan and lost 14.8 pounds of body fat and gained 7.9 pounds of lean muscle mass. Hank, at 76, was able to lose 9.3 pounds of body fat and gain 14.1 pounds of muscle mass. Such gains can become the norm when you follow this program. Serious resistance training can change the entire paradigm of aging.

The formula for stronger, more youthful mitochondria is straightforward:

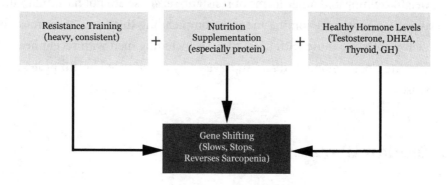

You're Never Too Old to Start Exercising

All men undergo a menopauselike phenomenon called andropause, an insidious, slow shift that affects hormonal levels and creates a heightened risk for chronic disease and death. When andropause hits, men as young as 40 begin to gain weight, lose muscle mass, become depressed, and experience low libido and often sexual performance issues. Most of all, they find that their energy levels diminish, creating self-esteem problems, a lowered sense of well-being, and reduced work productivity. Whatever you may be experiencing, exercise is the key to maintaining a higher-quality life and controlling the aging process. It's never too late to start—so you might as well start right now.

You might be thinking, "Is he crazy?" "I'm way too old," or, "I just can't do that." But as you've learned from my story, age is not a factor if you want to reclaim your life. As I became more comfortable with exercise, I realized that starting a rigorous program at my age was really not an issue. In fact, just the opposite is true. My exercise program can actually increase your level of fitness and health by 10 to 20 percent, decreasing your "biological age" by 10 to 20 years.

Doctors used to advise middle-aged and older men to get plenty of aerobic exercise: the constant rhythmic movements that increase heart rate for a sustained period of time. Walking, jogging, swimming, bicycle riding, and so on have always been thought to be the best exercise to help prevent or treat heart disease. What's more, doctors had traditionally discouraged men with heart disease from engaging in strength training because they believed it would put dangerous stress on their hearts.

But that myth was finally put to rest. The American Heart Association released data that show that weight training and other forms of resistance exercise are not harmful to the heart; doctors across the country are joining me in recommending this form of exercise for their healthy patients, as well as those with heart disease, including men with recent heart attacks, as long as they are closely monitored and supervised by experienced health professionals. So no more excuses!

The Life Plan Workouts

My Life Plan is different from any other exercise program because it focuses on three core exercise components, what I call the Mighty Three. If you do these types of exercise in combination throughout your week, you will see results quickly and continue with the program forever. I will give you the strategies that I have learned to make sure you can begin exercising at a level that is comfortable for you. Then, you'll learn how to follow the program, and stay on it, or get back on track when life gets in the way. Also, you'll be able to do all of these exercises and avoid injuries. You'll see how each of these types of exercise can improve your overall health, now and going forward.

- Balance, flexibility, and core strength

- Resistance training

- Cardio

Flexibility, Balance, and Core Strength
Keep You on Your Feet

A critical element in my physical fitness program is improving balance, or neuromuscular stabilization—which is the body's ability to slow down external resistance and stabilize the kinetic chain in all three planes of motion (that is, not falling down). The kinetic chain is the muscular, nervous, and joint systems all working together to create a fluid movement.

Improving balance through stretching and enhancing flexibility prevents injury. Your muscles can get to the most efficient level of strength if they are 1.2 times their resting length. Creating slightly elongated muscle means having a bigger range of motion. The longer your muscle is when it's resting, the more efficient it will be in the wider motion range. Better training plus more efficiency equals better body composition, more muscle mass, more strength, higher metabolism, more youthful appearance, better health, and more enjoyment out of your workout. Flexibility is also crucial for maintaining muscular strength, proper posture, full-range motion, and a spry, youthful gait.

My balance and flexibility program includes exercises tailored for men. You'll find that not only will they enhance your flexibility and balance, they will help reduce stress, alleviate low back pain, and diminish injury risks from your other physical activities. You'll learn more about all aspects of balance and flexibility in Chapter 5.

"In 2005, as I aided those in need during Hurricane Katrina with my organization, Corps of Compassion, my health began to deteriorate rapidly and seemingly without reason. My weight ballooned to over 250 pounds, my heaviest ever. It was a struggle to even make it through my daily activities because of the chronic fatigue, sleep disorders, major GI issues, and very low libido.

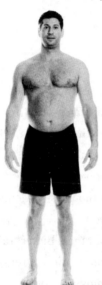

"I sought help from the very best practitioners I could find, including traditional doctors, Eastern medicine, and even homeopathic solutions. Unfortunately, nothing seemed to help. As fate would have it, I was introduced to Dr. Life. The conversation we had the first day I met him changed not only my health, but my life, forever. I was impressed by his knowledge, his skill, and his personal application. He walks his talk. I knew he was the right doctor for me.

"As soon as I began Dr. Life's program I noticed immediate results, like increased energy, fat loss, muscle tonality, increased libido, and overall enthusiasm for life again. Now, five years later, I'm 43 years old, and I look and feel better than I did when I was selected for a photo shoot as one of *People* magazine's "50 Hottest Bachelors" several years ago. As I continue my health journey with Dr. Life as my mentor, I am inspired to know with complete certainty that at *any* age, I can look and feel even better than in my youth. Thank you, Dr. Life, for changing my life and more important, my health, forever."

Resistance Training Builds Strong Muscles and Bones

"Just get moving" is traditional medicine's generic exercise prescription. While moving (I'm guessing they mean aerobic exercise) is important, you also have to start pushing yourself to new limits for muscle growth and adaptation. It's the only way to experience real health benefits. Your muscles are living entities, which are constantly using energy. That's where building muscle mass comes into play. It causes you to have a higher metabolism, so you are burning more calories even when you're not exercising.

Muscle and strength loss can be stopped and reversed only with resistance exercise. As our muscle mass increases, so does our strength. Having increased muscle mass and strength is the first step toward reversing physical frailty. Balance and coordination also improve with weight lifting, which reduces our chance of falling—a major source of injury, fractures, and debilitation leading to death for men as they age.

I believe that frailty is so important to prevent because most doctors are not addressing it correctly. When you go to see your primary care doctor, will a bone scan be part of your annual checkup? Probably not. Even if you ask for one, most insurance companies typically won't pay for a DEXA scan, even if risk factors are present. As a result, many men are walking around with serious bone issues and don't know it. According to the National Osteoporosis Foundation, 2 million men have osteoporosis and another 12 million are at risk, yet osteoporosis in men remains "underdiagnosed

THE BENEFITS OF INCREASING YOUR STRENGTH

1. Improves emotional state
2. Improves mental clarity
3. Enables us to have a more powerful presence
4. Enhances self-confidence
5. Extends to all areas of our personal and professional lives
6. Promotes increased production of our own hormones

and underreported." The disease causes 1.5 million fractures every year: 300,000 hip fractures, 250,000 wrist fractures, 700,000 vertebral fractures, and 300,000 other site fractures. The CDC states "approximately 20 percent of individuals with hip fractures will die the year after the fracture from surgery complications, such as pneumonia or blood clots in the lung."

In my practice, there isn't a week that goes by that I don't see a male patient who is osteopenic or osteoporotic. The good news is that things can be turned around with comprehensive diagnostics, correcting hormone deficiencies, the right nutrients (calcium, vitamin D3, and so on), and weight-bearing exercise.

Staying Aerobically Fit Equals More Independent Living

A significant study published in January 2008 found that men who were "highly fit" had a 50 to 70 percent lower mortality risk than their "low-fit" counterparts. According to the study, a regular exercise program can slow or reverse the loss of aerobic fitness, reducing the individual's biological age and prolonging independence. Progressive aerobic training can delay loss of independence by 10 to 12 years. The last thing any of us want is to have to depend on others to take care of us.

Aerobic exercise is particularly important for prevention of heart disease and for treatment after a heart attack, angioplasty, or bypass surgery. Just one session of aerobic activity can reduce blood pressure for up to 24 hours. When aerobic exercise is performed regularly, this effect—called postexercise hypotension—can decrease blood pressure by 5 to 7 mm Hg.

A study published in 2000 in the *New England Journal of Medicine* showed that in sedentary men, the endothelium (the lining of the blood vessels and heart) becomes more impaired as they get older. However, regular aerobic exercise can prevent age-related loss of endothelial function. And it can "restore damaged endothelium to healthy levels in previously sedentary middle-aged and older healthy men."

Doctors used to believe that it took weeks or months of regular exercise to gain any degree of protection for the heart. Yet new studies show that each exercise session stimulates the heart to increase its synthesis of protective proteins—stress proteins. Within 24 hours after exercising, these proteins increase enough to protect the heart against a variety of physical stresses. Moderate exercise can up your protection greatly. In fact, exercise intensity above that improves the protection gain by only a modest amount.

The most important lesson for cardio work is that you have to stay with it: Research shows that exercise-induced cardiac protection is lost once regular exercise is stopped. If you stop exercising, the synthesis of those protective proteins comes to a halt. In under a week, you'll be back to your pre-exercise level. No matter how long or how intensely you've been training, you'll be back to where you started in less than seven days, and you'll put your heart at risk.

On my Life Plan you will be doing some form of aerobic activity three to seven days a week. Aerobic exercise should involve continuous movement of your large muscle groups for 30 to 60 minutes or more in the range of "somewhat hard" to "hard." High-intensity interval training can dramatically shorten this time. You'll learn more about the specifics of this plan in Chapter 7.

Combining Aerobic Exercise with Resistance Training

Aerobic exercise and resistance training clearly work hand in hand to prevent, reduce, or even eliminate heart disease as they prevent or control diabetes, high cholesterol, and high blood pressure. Aerobic exercise does a great job lowering systolic blood pressure, and both aerobic and resistance exercise help reduce diastolic blood pressure. This makes it much easier for the heart to do its job of pumping blood throughout the body. Both forms of exercise also strengthen the heart muscle, making it work much more efficiently.

Dr. Kenneth Cooper now believes a mix of aerobic conditioning and strength training is the best exercise program for aging adults, because he recognizes, as I do, that as we age, we need more strength training. His exercise ratio protocol is as follows:

- Age 40 or younger: 80 percent aerobics and 20 percent strength training

- 41 to 50: 70/30

- 51 to 60: 60/40

- 61 and beyond: 55/45

I personally believe the ratio should be about 50/50 for just about everybody who wants to achieve and maintain great health, strength, and endurance. Strength training and cardio are just as important to a 40-year-old as to a 70-plus-year-old.

Exercise with a Coach or Personal Trainer

Some men are more successful with following—and staying on—an exercise program if they have a personal trainer. There are many advantages to having a personal trainer. Good trainers will take your training to heights you never dreamed possible. They will also prove to be invaluable as they:

- Teach proper form and technique

- Provide motivation

- Monitor progress

- Provide constructive criticism

- Provide positive reinforcement

- Provide an incentive (your accountability, their cost, or even better, their personality) to get to the gym

If you decide that a personal trainer would help you with your exercise program, it is important that you find one who has been certified and has proven that he or she has an understanding of physiology, exercise physiology, and exercise prescription. The top three organizations are known to offer a rigorous certification examination. You want your personal trainer to be certified by any one of these three:

- NSCA: The National Strength & Conditioning Association (requires a college degree)— www.nsca-lift.org

- ACE: The American Council on Exercise—www.acefitness.org

- ACSM: The American College of Sports Medicine—www.acsm.org

I believe that every man who can afford it should work with a trainer. I owe much of my success to my two trainers, Ernie Baul in Pennsylvania and Rod Stanley in Las Vegas. Ernie helped me win the Body-*for*-LIFE contest, and Rod has played a pivotal role in helping me increase my strength and muscle mass over the past four years. These guys have made resistance training fun and challenging for me and have inspired me to get up early and get my butt to the gym.

Do I Need Sports Drinks?

Over the last few years there have been an increasing number of sports drinks on the supermarket shelves that claim to provide not only fluid, but also essential nutrients that will improve muscle strength, endurance, and overall performance. The truth is, there is nothing magical about any of these beverages. They all contain carbohydrates, which have been clearly shown to be beneficial during exercise—when muscle glycogen levels are near depletion and blood glucose levels are low.

Research has shown, however, that carbohydrate ingestion is beneficial only during prolonged exercise. If pre-exercise nutrition is adequate, there is no need to ingest carbohydrates during continuous exercise lasting less than 90 minutes. In fact, when we ingest carbohydrates during short-term exercise, it simply increases the calories we take in and interferes with our efforts to get rid of body fat.

As far as electrolytes are concerned, only small amounts are lost when you sweat during very heavy exercise, and these can easily be replaced by eating fruits or vegetables later in the day. Only endurance athletes who sweat heavily for extended periods need to replenish their electrolytes while exercising.

However, you do need to drink lots of water when you are exercising. Drink more than you think you need. People are notorious for underestimating the amount of water they require.

MOTIVATORS FOR EXERCISE

1. Exercise with a friend. Statistics tell us that people who exercise with a friend are more successful at staying with their program. Knowing that someone is waiting for you can be great motivation to show up and get it done!

2. Train for an event, like a local 5k or 10k walk or run in your area. I've seen many men transformed from couch potatoes to lean, mean, exercising machines because they decided to enter and train for a competition. Just look at me: Don't think you can't do it . . . YOU CAN!

3. Reward yourself! Find a nonfood item that you can use as a reward. I'm sure there's something at your local electronics store that you have your eye on.

4. Keep records. Write down your exercise time each day. Keep a running total for a week, month, and year. Calculate your average exercise time per day. Set some lofty goals!

Keep Breathing

For all of the Life Plan Workouts, it's important to maintain proper breathing. Always—even when you are just walking around—breathe in through your nose and out through your mouth. The nose is the primary way we breathe in clean, heated, and filtered air, so if you breathe through your mouth, you are taking in air that is not perfectly treated for your body. Breathe from your diaphragm by allowing your belly to extend, instead of your chest, on every inhalation; your belly should draw in during every exhalation.

During your cardio workouts it's important to continue to remain relaxed. You can accomplish this by breathing deeply and slowly and avoiding shallow breaths. Concentrate on your breathing and keep it well controlled.

During martial arts or other flexibility and balance exercises, it's critical that you not hold your breath. Breath control is one of the important skills men learn during their martial arts training.

During the resistance training workouts, never hold your breath, because this increases your blood pressure and can cause a stroke. Instead, exhale when you are performing work or producing force against the weight or external resistance. Inhale when reducing force or slowing the weight or external resistance.

Get Moving!

- -

Now that you understand why you'll be exercising, look over the next three chapters to learn the program. Each of the Mighty Three has a different point of entry, depending on what your current fitness levels are: basic health, fitness, and high performance.

CHAPTER 5

The Life Plan Flexibility, Core, and Balance Workouts

Before I started training in the martial arts, I had never given flexibility or balance much thought. I just figured that as long as I was doing cardio and lifting weights consistently, I was taking care of my body. When I got stiff in my lower back, hips, and legs, which was pretty often, I just assumed that would improve with more strength training and cardio. But as my martial arts skills progressed and I was asked to start kicking my legs above my knees, I realized just how inflexible I was, and how prone I was to falling.

Flexibility is the ability to move all the joints—your fingers, hands, wrists, elbows, knees, hips, feet, toes, neck, and spine—freely through a full range of motion and without pain. I have found that the more flexible my joints are the less joint pain I have. Flexibility is like bone density and muscle mass: It's a "use it or lose it" situation. In order to "use it" you need to be able to comfortably twist, bend, turn, and reach. The flexibility exercises outlined in this chapter involve stretching, which teaches your body to move without restraint so that you will prevent muscular pain.

Loss of flexibility can also lead to balance problems. Tight muscles and joints—the cause of inflexibility—put undue stress on the joints and force the body into faulty movement patterns, lousy posture, and overall instability. When your body is forced to deal with muscle tightness, it sends distorted signals to your brain from your sensory nervous system, which triggers your body to compensate and recruit other muscles to perform a particular movement. For example, if your chest is tight it will cause your shoulders to round, making it impossible for your body to properly align and throwing you off balance.

All of the systems related to balance decline with aging if we let them. These include touch and pressure sensation on the bottoms of the feet, vision (both acuity and edge detection), proprioception (sensory information that provides feedback to your brain about joint position and movement), and vestibular input (the sense of body movement located in our inner ear). A loss of strength also affects balance. The muscle loss called sarcopenia, which I discussed in Chapter 4, is a major factor in the overall loss of balance and flexibility and greatly increases your risk of falls, fractures, and admission to nursing homes.

However, when you combine flexibility exercises with balance training, you create a win-win situation that will keep you from feeling old. The benefits of flexibility and balance training include:

- A more youthful gait

- Improved coordination

- Improved posture

- Improved reaction time

- Improved sexual function

- Increased range of motion

- Reduced lower back pain

- Reduced muscle soreness

- Reduced risk of muscle injury

- Reduced risk of falling

A FLEXIBLE MAN IS A SEXUAL MAN

Active vigorous sexual function is like any other athletic activity—the more strength, endurance, and flexibility you have the better you are at it. You can have great erectile function, but if you lack strength and endurance and your joints don't move very well, you will fail as a lover.

The Life Plan Flexibility Workout

In this book I have included two flexibility modalities: Self Myofascial Release (SMR), which should be done *before* resistance training *after* you have performed a brief cardio warmup, and Static Stretching, which should be completed *after* your total workout is done. You will be performing all of the flexibility exercises listed to ensure you have a comprehensive stretching program.

Self Myofascial Release

Fascia is the soft-tissue portion of the connective tissues and provides support for most tissues in the body, including the muscles. This soft tissue can become restricted due to trauma, injury, overuse, or inactivity, causing pain and tension. It can also limit the ability of the muscles to have proper blood flow. As in most tissue, irritation causes localized inflammation, which also leads to pain. Worse, chronic inflammation results in fibrosis, or the thickening of the connective tissue, and results in reflexive muscle tension that causes even more pain and inflammation. Myofascial techniques aim to break this cycle.

The technique I use for myofascial release is called "foam rolling" and requires that you purchase a foam roller at any sporting goods store. You will then place the foam roller under each muscle group until a tender area is found, and maintain pressure on the tender area for 30 to 60 seconds. This will result in releasing the fascia and softening and lengthening the muscle. It will help break down scar tissue and allow the muscles to reach optimal levels of lengthening during exercise.

You will complete each of the following nine positions with the foam roller, holding each one for 30 seconds. If you experience muscle tightness during any of these, repeat that position for an additional 30 to 60 seconds.

Inner thigh

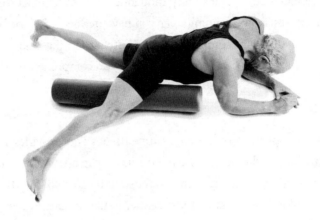

Calves

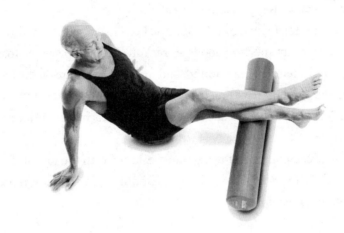

Back (upper)

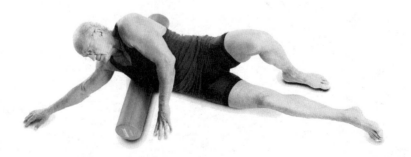

Quadriceps

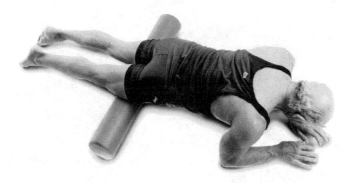

Outer leg (lying on side)

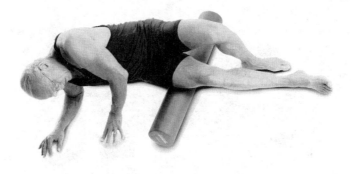

Hamstring

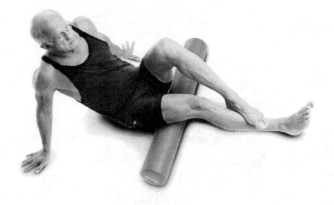

Peroneals (lower leg)

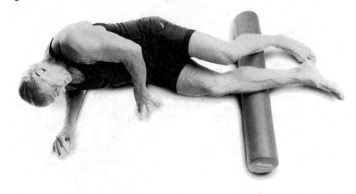

Midback

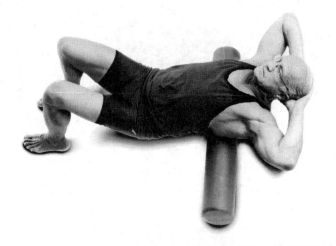

Gluteus

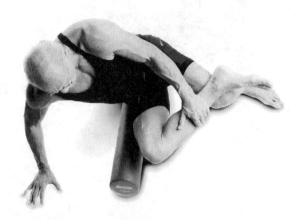

Static Stretching

This program is designed to stretch each of the major muscle groups so that you will be able to take each joint through its full range of motion. These exercises are best done after completing both your resistance training and your cardio workouts. If you have chronic muscle pain or stiffness in a particular area, such as the lower back, you will need to make sure that you complete those stretches that target that area at least three times a week. For example, I stretch my hamstrings and hip flexors every day.

Each of the following static stretch positions should be held for 20 to 30 seconds and then repeated with a complete relaxation of the muscle between repetitions. The stretches should be done in a gentle and relaxed motion, moving just to the point where you can feel a stretch in the muscles you are working, and not in the other muscles that you are not working. For example, if you are stretching your calves, you should not feel a pull in your back. Do not bounce during stretching.

Be patient during your stretches and do not force joints to go farther than they want. Severe pain while stretching is a signal that the stretch has gone too far. Mild to moderate pain during a stretch indicates you are doing the stretch properly to make advances. There should be no soreness the next day after a stretching routine; if there is, it is an indication that you have overstretched and should lower the intensity of stretching the next time you perform the exercises. This can be done by not stretching the muscle so far or by not holding the stretch as long.

Breathe slowly and never hold your breath while stretching. Proper breathing helps to relax your body, increases blood flow throughout your body, and helps to mechanically remove lactic acid and other by-products of exercise.

CORRECT POSTURE DEVIATIONS

For optimum balance and neuromuscular efficiency, you need to work continually at achieving good posture, muscle balance, flexibility, core stabilization, and good strength throughout your body. The best ways to correct postural deviations is by using a combination of static flexibility exercises and Self Myofascial Release (SMR). If you continue to train your body without correcting postural deviations it will be impossible to perform exercises with proper technique. Worse, it will increase your likelihood of getting injured.

NECK STRETCH

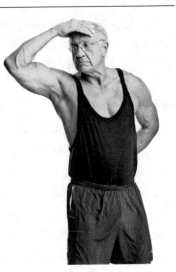

To start: Begin by standing with feet shoulder width apart.

1. Take your right hand and place it on the left side of your forehead just above the eyebrow.

2. Place the left arm behind your back with your hand in the middle of your back while rolling your left shoulder back.

3. Applying slight pressure, turn your head to the right until you feel a stretch on the left side of the neck.

4. Hold for 20 to 30 seconds, then rest and repeat on the other side.

LAT STRETCH

Benefits: Stretches the lateral muscles of your back.

To start: Stand with feet shoulder width apart.

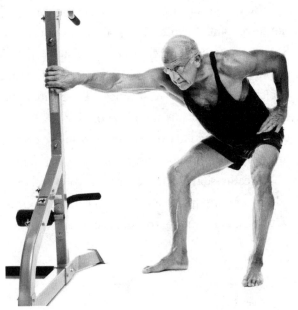

1. Grab a sturdy fixed object or doorway with the hand closest to your support object.

2. Lean forward at the waist, keeping your back straight.

3. Shift your weight away from the support until you feel a stretch in your lateral muscles.

4. Hold for 20 to 30 seconds and repeat on the other side.

SHOULDER STRETCH

Benefits: Stretches rear shoulder muscle.

To start: Stand with feet shoulder width apart, knees slightly bent, and toes pointed forward.

1. Place your left arm across your body at shoulder height and gently pull it toward your right shoulder with your right hand.

2. Continue holding your left arm either above or below the elbow.

3. Look over your left shoulder to deepen the stretch.

4. Hold for 20 to 30 seconds, then rest and repeat on the other side.

CHEST/SHOULDER GIRDLE STRETCH

Benefits: Stretches the chest and shoulders.

To start: Stand at the end of a sturdy fixed object or doorway with arm parallel to the floor.

1. Extend your arm and have only a slight bend in the elbow.

2. Turn your body away from your fixed object or doorway until you feel a stretch in the shoulders and pectoral or chest muscles.

3. Hold for 20 to 30 seconds and repeat on the other side.

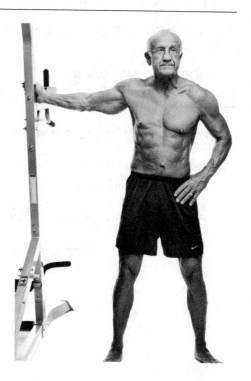

THORACIC SPINE STRETCH

Benefits: Stretches the muscles of the midback.

To start: Kneel on the floor on all fours with your knees under your hips and hands under your shoulders.

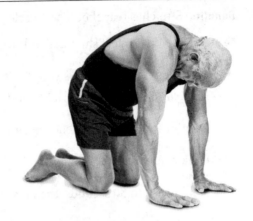

1. Keeping your palms flat on the floor, contract your abs to bring your head, neck, and back in alignment.

2. Tilt the hip bones toward the ceiling while drawing your shoulders back and down.

3. Tuck the chin in and round your back until you feel a stretch down your spine.

4. Hold for 20 to 30 seconds, then relax and repeat.

LOWER BACK STRETCH

Benefits: Stretches the lower back muscles.

To start: Lie on your back with your knees bent and feet flat on the floor.

1. Place both hands on top of your right shin, just below the knee, and gently pull your knee up into your chest.

2. For a deeper stretch, straighten your left leg out along the floor.

3. Hold for 20 to 30 seconds, then rest and repeat on the other side.

ABDOMINAL STRETCH

Benefits: Stretches the abdominal muscles. (This is good to do after performing an ab workout that causes the muscle to tighten. It's also great for increasing flexibility if you have a lower extremity postural distortion called "posterior pelvic tilt." Signs of this are tight abs and tight glutes.)

To start: Lie on your stomach with your legs straight behind you and palms on the floor directly underneath your chest.

1. Slowly straighten your elbows, then puff your chest out.

2. Slightly tilt your head up until you feel a stretch along your abs.

3. Hold for 20 to 30 seconds, then return to a lying position before repeating.

HIP FLEXOR STRETCH

Benefits: Stretches the hip flexors.

To start: Stand with your right leg forward and left leg back.

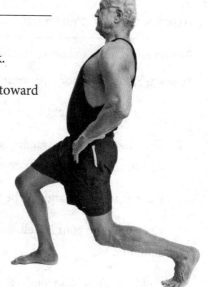

1. Keep your torso erect and slightly point your left foot toward your right foot.

2. Keep your left foot on the floor. Push your hips forward, allowing your right knee to bend.

3. Hold for 20 to 30 seconds and repeat on the other side.

QUAD STRETCH

Benefits: Stretches the quadriceps, the large muscles located on the front of the leg.

To start: Lie on a mat facedown and place your left hand between your forehead and the floor.

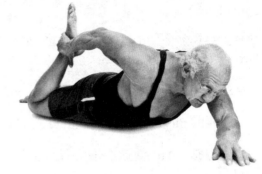

1. Keeping hips on the floor, bring your right leg up behind you and grab your foot.

2. Keep your head down and neck relaxed.

3. Hold for 20 to 30 seconds and repeat with left leg.

OUTER THIGH STRETCH

Benefits: Stretches the outer thigh and lower back.

To start: Sit on the floor with your left leg straight out in front of you and your right leg bent.

1. Cross your bent right leg over the left and place your right foot flat on the floor.

2. Keeping your back straight, gently press your left elbow against your outer right thigh and slowly twist your upper body to the right.

3. Place your right hand on the floor behind you, fingertips facing away from your body.

4. Keep pressing your left elbow into your right leg and slowly look over your right shoulder.

5. Hold for 20 to 30 seconds, then rest and repeat on the other side.

ADDUCTOR STRETCH

Benefits: Stretches the muscles of the inner thigh.

To start: Stand with your legs slightly wider than shoulder width apart, feet pointed straight ahead.

1. Shift your weight onto your left leg while bending the knee, keeping your right leg extended.

2. Rotate upper body in direction of left leg until stretch is felt in inner thigh of the right leg.

3. Hold for 20 to 30 seconds, then rest and repeat on the other side.

CALF STRETCH

Benefits: Stretches the calves.

To start: Stand with one leg behind you, keeping both feet flat on the floor and your rear knee straight.

1. Lean slightly forward until you feel tension in the calf of the extended leg. You may also place your hands on a wall for support.

2. Hold for 20 to 30 seconds and repeat on the other side.

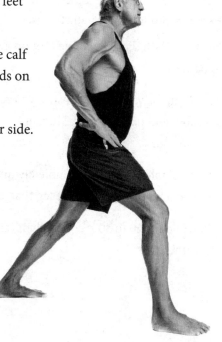

PIRIFORMIS STRETCH

Benefits: Stretches the piriformis, the muscle located on the upper part of the buttocks. It is part of the lateral rotators of the hip and is tight in almost everybody who doesn't actively stretch it on a regular basis.

To start: Lie on your back. Place your right ankle on your left knee.

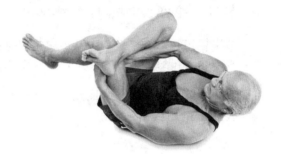

1. Keep your head on the floor while you reach around the left thigh.

2. Pull both legs toward you as you push on your right knee with your right hand or elbow.

3. Hold for 20 to 30 seconds and repeat on opposite side.

HAMSTRING STRETCH

Benefits: Stretches the hamstrings.

To start: Place the heel of one foot on a sturdy apparatus.

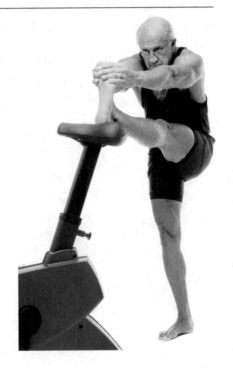

1. Lean forward at the waist as you reach to grab one foot and pull it forward in front on you.

2. Straighten both legs completely until you feel the stretch in the back of the leg that is in the air.

3. Hold for 20 to 30 seconds, then repeat on the other side.

Core/Abdominal Training

The core consists of muscles in the lower back, hips, pelvis, and the abdominals. Having a strong core is like building a strong foundation for a house. A house with a weak foundation cannot withstand the conditions that it has to face year after year. Similarly, if you have a weak core you will not withstand the demands of day-to-day activities. Having a weak core affects your overall fitness level, athletic performance, and sexual performance. Having an efficient core allows your body to maintain correct postural alignment while training and helps your body stabilize in the face of other external forces. The ability to maintain proper body alignment during everyday movement and athletic activities will significantly reduce your risk for injury.

On this program you will be performing some core work each time you exercise. Depending on which program you follow, you will be choosing 2 to 3 exercises from the following.

ABS/CORE CRUNCH

Benefits: Strengthens the abdominals.

To start: Lie with your back pressing against the floor. Place your hands loosely behind your head, knees bent, feet flat on the floor. Do not pull on your neck. Look up to the ceiling. Imagine that you have placed a tennis ball underneath your chin.

1. Begin to curl your upper body 2 inches off the floor.

2. Contract your abdominal muscles on the way up by bringing your rib cage toward your pelvis. Do not let your shoulder blades touch the floor.

3. Perform 20 to 25 repetitions per set.

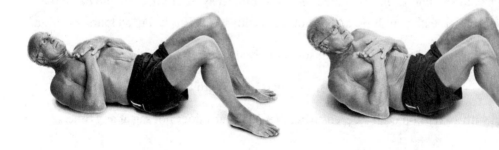

PLANK

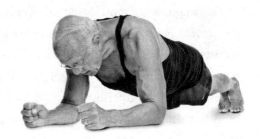

Benefits: Strengthens the core.

To start: Assume a modified pushup position, on your forearms and toes. Your body will form a straight line from your shoulders to your ankles.

1. Pull your abs in but don't stick out your butt.

2. Hold this position with a straight body for 2 to 3 minutes.

SIDE PLANK

Benefits: Strengthens the core.

To start: Lie on your side. Lift up your body while facing forward and support your weight on the forearm and the outside edge of your foot. Keep your elbow directly underneath your shoulder. Your body will form a straight line from your shoulders to your ankles.

1. Pull in your abs and keep your body in a straight line.

2. Hold this position for at least 20 seconds.

OPPOSITE ARM LEG REACH

Benefits: Strengthens the core.

To start: Position your body on a mat or the floor, placing the palms of your hands directly underneath your shoulders, and straighten the arms completely. Your knees should be on the floor directly underneath your hips, about shoulder width apart. This is the "all fours" position.

1. Extend one leg and the opposite arm so that they are parallel to the floor.

2. Hold this position for 3 to 4 seconds, and then repeat with the opposite arm and leg.

3. Begin with 10 reps on each side, ensuring that your back does not sag at any time.

BICYCLE CRUNCH

Benefits: Strengthens the abdominals.

To start: Lie on your back on the floor with your hands loosely behind your head. Raise your legs to form a 90-degree angle at your knees.

1. Curl your upper body and crunch your abdominal muscles, bringing your left elbow toward your right side while drawing your right knee in to meet it.

2. Continue to alternate sides, back and forth, for a total of 15 times per set.

SUPERMANS

Benefits: Strengthens the core.

To start: Lie facedown on the floor with your ankles flexed and your toes on the floor.

1. Extend your arms on the floor out to your sides in a T position with your thumbs facing up.

2. Pressing your shoulder blades down and back, lift your arms perpendicular to your body, forming a T shape. Hold position for 1 to 2 minutes. Return to the starting position and rest.

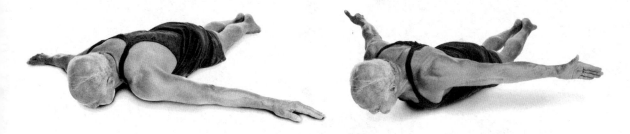

BALL REVERSE CRUNCH

Benefits: This exercise will work the abdominals.

To start: Ensure that you have a steady surface to hold on to (a bench or rail, for example). Lie down with your back on an exercise ball. The ball should be around the middle of the back.

1. Reach overhead to grasp your steady surface, then keep your legs bent at a 90-degree angle.

2. Rotate your hips and pelvis forward until your knees touch your chest.

3. Slowly lower your legs to starting position. Complete 20 to 25 per set.

NOTE: Stop immediately if you feel pain in your lower back.

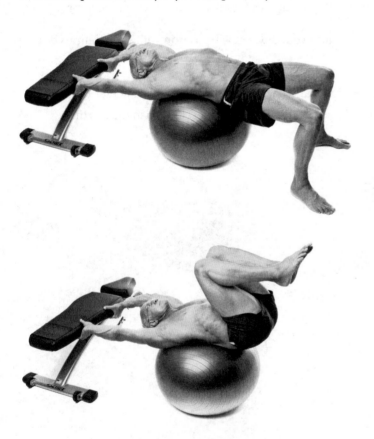

ADVANCED CABLE TRUNK ROTATION

Benefits: Core-strengthening exercise.

To start: Begin with feet shoulder width apart. Grasp a single cable handle with both hands.

1. Rotate the trunk of your body away from the cable pulley.

2. Rotate until the hip, knee, and ankle are all extended.

3. Return to starting position with feet shoulder width apart.

4. Begin with 10 repetitions for both sides.

PLANK OPPOSITE-ARM-LEG REACH

Benefits: Exercise will improve core strength.

To start: Assume a modified pushup position, on your forearms and toes. Your body will form a straight line from your shoulders to your ankles. Pull your abs in but don't stick out your butt.

1. Extend your right arm straight in front of you until your arm is completely straight.

2. Lift your left leg off the floor about 5 inches. Hold for 20 seconds.

3. Return to original position and repeat with left arm and right leg.

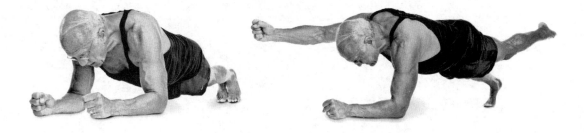

BALL KNEE TUCK WITH ROTATION

Benefits: Exercise will improve core strength.

To start: Begin by placing both hands on an exercise ball in a pushup position.

1. While keeping hands on the ball, extend arms to a locked-elbow position. Draw abdominals in and bring one knee in toward the exercise ball.

2. When your knees and hips are flexed at a 90-degree angle, rotate your knee underneath your body by twisting your torso.

3. Return to starting position. Repeat 10 on each side per set.

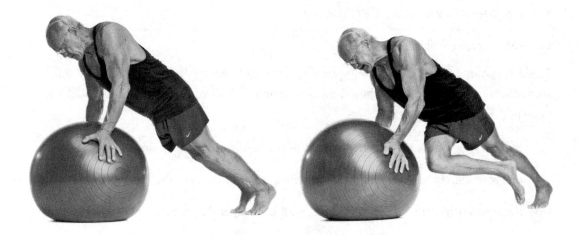

Advanced Flexibility Workout

You can continue to improve your flexibility by extending the duration of each stretch, the intensity of the stretch, the velocity of the movement, and the frequency with which you perform the movements.

Once you have corrected any posture deviations you might have—and you're able to take each joint through its full range of motion—you can start incorporating some active flexibility into your training program. We don't just move along a straight path. We twist, turn, cut corners, bend over, and pick things up. Therefore, it's important to include exercises that extend your joints through their full range of motion and in all planes of motion—such as Pilates, walking lunges with rotation, pushups with rotation, and martial arts.

WALKING KNEE GRABS

Benefits: This exercise will stretch the glute muscles and warm up your entire body.

To start: Stand erect with feet together.

1. Take one step with your left leg while grabbing your right knee up in front of you, pulling it as high as you can while extending the rest of your body. Think about staying tall.

2. Repeat on the other side. Keep traveling forward with each stretch until you've done 10 reps with each leg.

WALKING QUAD STRETCH

Benefits: This exercise will stretch the quadriceps and warm up your entire body.

To start: Stand erect with feet together.

1. Take one step forward with your left leg while bending the right knee back and grabbing the right ankle until a stretch is felt in the front of the right leg.

2. Hold stretch for 3 to 5 seconds and release.

3. Repeat on other side until you have completed 10 repetitions on each side.

Benefits: This exercise will stretch your thighs, hips, and buttocks.

To start: Stand alongside a wall. Place one hand on the wall.

1. Draw your navel inward.

2. Swing your right leg forward, with control, while your left arm touches your right leg.

3. Swing leg backward. Keep midsection tight.

4. Repeat on left leg.

5. Complete 10 repetitions on each leg.

Real Men Do Pilates

I had been working on my flexibility for over a year before I made significant progress. One day, when I was struggling with my stretching exercises at the gym, I happened to see someone working out on a strange-looking apparatus. I learned that it was called a Pilates Reformer, and it was specifically designed to stretch the body in ways I never dreamed possible.

The Pilates machine and floor exercise technique were developed by trainer/gymnast Joseph Pilates in 1926. His principles of exercise centered on postural muscles, which result in better balance, support, flexibility, longer/leaner muscles, and agility. This method of conditioning was initially called Contrology. Over the course of his career, he developed more than 600 exercises for various pieces of apparatus he invented. His equipment is designed to condition the entire body, using positions and movements that duplicate functional activities, which help improve body alignment and posture by improving balance, strength, flexibility, and coordination. Pilates targets stiff muscles and joints while enhancing core strength at the same time.

Today, Pilates is one of the fastest-growing exercise methods in the world. The exercises emphasize an awareness of proper breathing and the right spinal/pelvic alignment. His workouts are performed either on a mat using your body as the weight or on other resistance-based equipment such as the Pilates Reformer (a sliding platform), Pilates Chair (used for sculpting/toning legs, arms, buttocks, and thighs), Pilates Cadillac (a large unit with trapeze, horizontal bar), and many others.

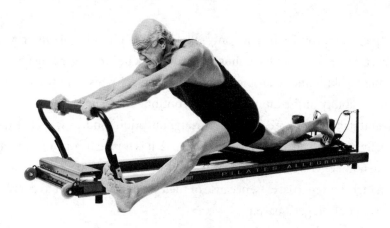

For the past three years, I have worked on Pilates machines for one hour, three times a week. I have found that this has dramatically improved my posture, flexibility, gait, and agility. It is by far the fastest way I have found to improve flexibility and balance. Today I move faster and more youthfully than I did in my 30s. I really have become a believer that whatever your fitness level, you can begin a body-conditioning Pilates program that will help protect you from injuries, greatly improve your flexibility, and increase your strength. For more information about Pilates programs in your area, visit www.pilatesmethodalliance.org.

Martial Arts

I had been intrigued by martial arts for some time, even before my formal training began. I started training in Tae Kwon Do when I moved to Las Vegas eight years ago and am now in pursuit of a black belt. One of the major reasons I like Tae Kwon Do so much is that it demands total concentration. For a few hours each week I can block out all the pressures of my daily life. It requires focus, clarity of mind, inner peace, self-respect, respect for others, and discipline. I have found that it has greatly improved my overall motor skills, muscle memory, and quick reaction time.

Martial arts require flexibility, balance, speed, and coordination—the very things that are lost as men age. In conjunction with my complete Life Plan, including strength training, cardiovascular endurance, low-glycemic/low-fat nutrition, and correcting my hormonal deficiencies, Tae Kwon Do has helped me at age 72 do many of the things a 20-something has trouble doing. I strongly believe that martial arts have been integral to my successful healthy aging. While I'm no street fighter—and probably will never be (but who knows?)—I've definitely moved way beyond my father's concept of aging.

For example, Tae Kwon Do has not only enhanced my physique, it's improved my cognitive fitness. Several recent studies have shown a strong link between learning new and complex physical and mental skills and neuroplasticity. Neuroplasticity, also known as cortical remapping, refers to the ability of the human brain to continue to change and grow. We now know that the brain and its functions are not fixed throughout adulthood, as was once thought. Your brain can actually rewire itself, making you smarter, as it is forced to adapt to new and complex physical and mental activities. In other words, your brain's physical anatomy and physiology can actually change, and martial arts, because of their focus on attention to detail, are one way that you can help yourself get smarter.

The value of martial arts training for me far exceeds my ability to master the intricate steps, footwork, kicking, jumping, blocking, and punching that I've learned as I have moved through the ranks. I believe that the overall philosophy of pushing oneself beyond personal limits, which is interwoven in all martial arts, applies to every facet of life. It is a large part of how I can keep focused on a healthy path. Tae Kwon Do and most of the other martial arts enable you to dig deep within yourself and discover an inner power—which is referred to as your "indomitable spirit"—that helps you to unite your mind and body for an unstoppable attitude about anything you decide to accomplish.

The Life Plan Balance Workout

Improving your balance requires very little extra time out of your day. Balance training should be systematic, progressive, and functional, so begin with the exercises that fit your particular balance level and work your way into the more advanced levels. You will be performing one or two of these exercises every time you train. There are three types of balance exercises, so mix them up as you see fit.

TEST YOUR ABILITY TO BALANCE

The first step toward improving your balance is to determine your current balance level. The following are some tests you can do at home. If you think your ability to balance is compromised, have someone close by watch you complete these. Time yourself to accurately document how long you were able to hold the position.

- Single leg reach—stand on one leg with eyes opened or closed and extend your nonsupporting leg to the front, side, or back. Hold that position for as long as you can.

- Stork test—standing with your arms out to your sides, bringing the bottom of one foot to the inside knee of the other leg and hold that position with eyes opened or closed for as long as you can.

Traditional Balance Exercises

STEP UP BALANCE

Benefits: Improves balance, stability, and core strength.

To start: Stand in front of a step or box with your feet shoulder width apart.

1. Step onto the step with your right leg.

2. Lift your left leg until your upper leg is parallel to the floor.

3. Step down with both legs.

4. Repeat steps 1 to 3 for 10 to 20 repetitions, switching legs each time.

Benefits: Improves balance, stability, and core strength.

To start: Stand with your feet shoulder width apart. It's a good idea to perform this exercise near a wall or piece of equipment in case you lose your balance.

1. Slowly lift one leg off the floor, at a minimum of 6 inches. Hold this position for about 30 seconds.

2. Lower your leg to the floor.

3. Repeat 10 to 20 times, switching sides each time.

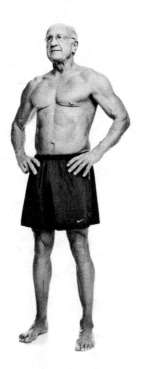
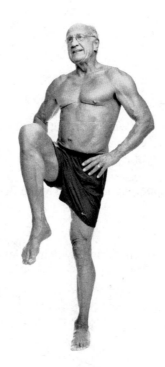

SINGLE LEG REACH

Benefits: Improves balance, stability, and core strength.

To start: Stand with your feet shoulder width apart. It's a good idea to perform this exercise near a wall or piece of equipment in case you lose your balance.

1. Lift one leg about 6 inches off the floor.

2. Extend the leg that is off the floor in front of you.

3. Return to starting position.

4. Repeat 10 to 20 times for each leg.

For variation you can extend the leg to the side or behind you while standing on the other leg.

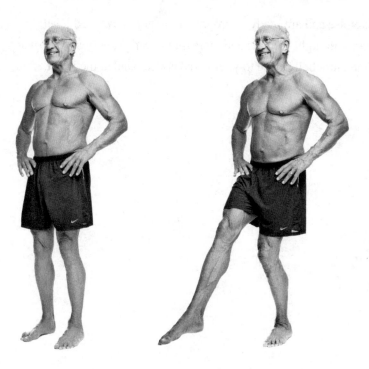

SINGLE LEG DEAD LIFT

Benefits: Improves balance, stability, and core strength.

To start: Stand with your feet shoulder width apart. It's a good idea to perform this exercise near a wall or piece of equipment in case you lose your balance.

1. Lift one leg in the air about 6 inches off the floor.

2. Lean forward at the waist, keeping your back straight.

3. Continue to bend at the waist until your upper body is parallel with the floor.

4. Return to starting position.

5. Repeat 10 to 20 times with each leg.

When you have mastered this exercise and are ready to progress to a more advanced level, you can hold two dumbbells. Start with light weights and increase the weight very slowly over several weeks. Be sure to keep the dumbbells close to your body as you bend at the waist.

Benefits: Improves balance, stability, and core strength.

To start: Stand with your feet shoulder width apart. It's a good idea to perform this exercise near a wall or piece of equipment in case you lose your balance. It's okay to hold on to a railing or sturdy support while performing this exercise.

1. Lift one leg about 6 inches off the floor.

2. Lower your body to the floor by bending the knee of the planted leg and keeping the opposite leg off the floor.

3. Continue to squat until the planted leg reaches a 45-degree angle.

4. Return to starting position.

5. Repeat 10 to 20 times with each leg.

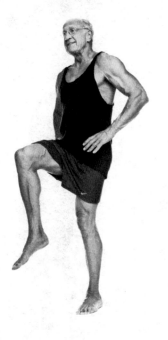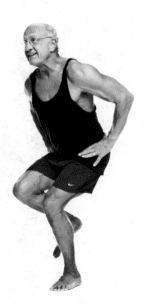

Advanced Balance Workout

The following techniques are more advanced and should be used by those who have an above-average level of balance or are committed to spending additional time on improving their balance. You can practice any of the above listed techniques while closing your eyes, or try using an unstable platform such as a Dyna disc or BOSU ball. These can be found at your local gym or purchased for home use.

BOSU BALL DUMBBELL OVERHEAD PRESS

Benefits: Improves balance, stability, and core strength and strengthens shoulders.

To start: Stand with your feet shoulder width apart on a BOSU ball with two dumbbells.

1. Bring two dumbbells to shoulder height with your upper arms parallel to the floor.

2. Press the weights directly overhead until your arms are fully extended.

3. Return to the starting position. Upper arm (triceps) should remain parallel to the floor.

4. Perform 8 to 12 repetitions.

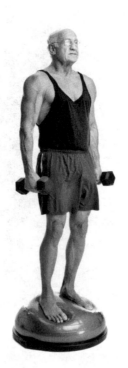
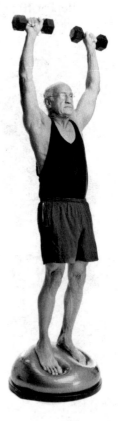

BOSU BALL TRICEPS EXTENSION

Benefits: Improves balance, stability, and core strength and strengthens triceps.

To start: Stand with your feet shoulder width apart on a BOSU ball with two dumbbells. Bend at the waist, so your upper body is not quite parallel to the floor. Your knees should be slightly bent, with your back straight.

1. Keeping your upper arms alongside your body, extend your elbows at a 90-degree angle.

2. Slowly extend your arms and contract your triceps at the top of the movement.

3. Return to the starting position.

4. Repeat 8 to 12 times.

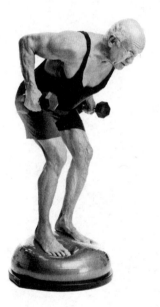 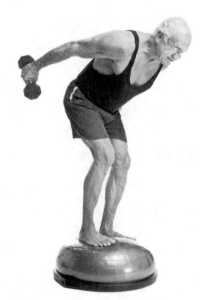

SINGLE LEG, BOSU BALL CURL

Benefits: Stabilization exercise for biceps.

To start: Stand on a BOSU ball with one leg. Hold a dumbbell in each hand.

1. Curl the dumbbell up, both arms at the same time, toward your chest in a slow, controlled manner.

2. Contract your biceps at the top of the movement.

3. Slowly lower the dumbbells to the original starting position.

4. Repeat 8 to 12 times.

Functional Training Improves Balance

You can easily enhance balance and joint stability with exercises that mimic everyday life, which are referred to as *functional training*. A good functional-training program will involve exercises that move your body in all four planes of motion: forward, backward, rotational, and lateral. An example of functional training is bending over to pick something up off the floor and putting it on a shelf. This can easily be simulated by picking up a dumbbell from the floor and pressing it overhead. Each of these excercises should be repeated 20 to 25 times per set.

- Elastic Band Trunk Rotation: rotating the trunk, which causes you to work in the transverse plane.

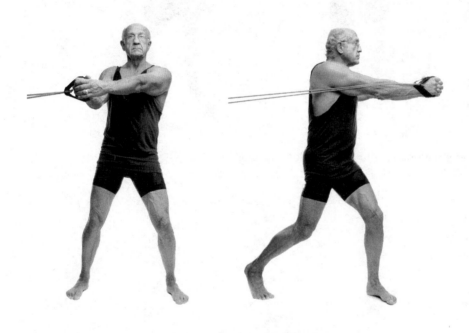

- Medicine Ball Press: picking up a medicine ball, pressing it either in front of you or above your head, and placing it back on the floor.

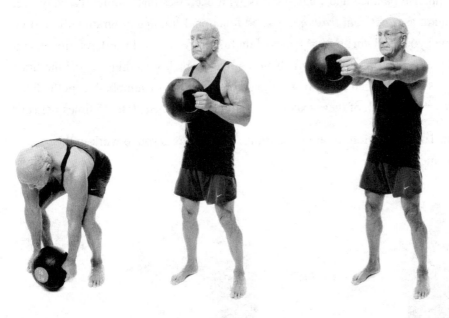

- Side Lunge: strengthens your body's lateral motion.

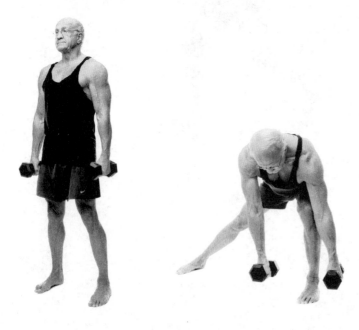

ICE SKATERS WITH TOE TOUCH

Benefits: Improves balance, stability, and core strength.

To start: Stand with your feet shoulder width apart in a slightly squatting position.

1. Pushing off with the left leg, jump to the right side, landing on the right leg, in a squatting position.

2. As you land softly, twist at the waist to touch your right toe with your left hand.

3. Repeat in a continuous motion for 20 to 30 seconds, alternating right and left legs.

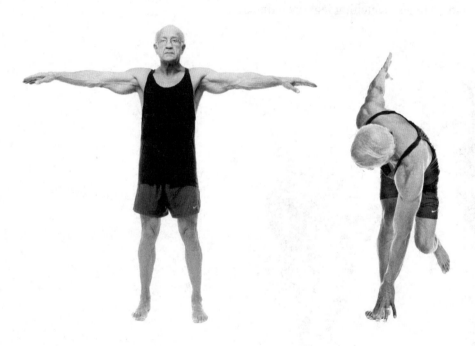

Benefits: Improves balance, stability, and core strength.

To start: Stand with your feet shoulder width apart. It's a good idea to perform this exercise near a wall or piece of equipment in case you lose your balance.

1. Lift your right leg off the floor 6 inches.

2. Lean forward at the waist and touch your left foot with your right hand.

3. Return to starting position.

4. Repeat 10 to 20 times, switching legs each time.

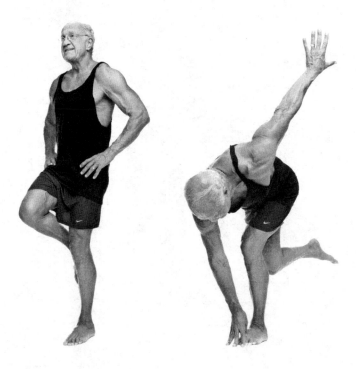

On-the-Go Balance Training

The following is a list of simple ways to improve balance that you can do anytime, anywhere.

1. Walk through your house as if you were walking on a tightrope. Walk by placing the toe of one foot touching the heel of the other, then place the lagging foot at the toe of the front foot. Repeat until you reach your destination. You can also do this outside on a curb.

2. Figure 8 walking. Walk in a figure 8 more and more quickly, with the 8 getting smaller and smaller.

3. Stand on one foot for at least 30 seconds. A good goal is at least 60 seconds per foot. Keep track so you can see how you progress each month.

4. Balance on one leg while performing daily activities (brushing your teeth, cooking, showering, or combing your hair). Remember to keep your knee slightly bent.

5. Pick up objects (newspaper, shoes, pen, and so on) while standing on one leg. This may not sound very hard, but be sure to have something nearby to hold on to in case you fall.

STRENGTH TRAINING IMPROVES BALANCE

Focus your strength-training program to include exercises for the muscles in the hips, glutes, low back, abdominals, and core if you are already experiencing problems with balance.

CHAPTER 6

The Life Plan Resistance Training Workouts

Our bodies tend to lose muscle mass and gain body fat as we get older. Resistance training is really the key to turning that trend around. It is the single most effective way to lose body fat and achieve a high level of strength, muscle mass, and physical fitness. Yet while many men are intrigued by resistance training, I find that they are fearful or hesitant at the same time. I can tell you firsthand that without resistance training I would never look or feel as good as I do. And while I do get sore from time to time after a good workout, I never train to the point of injury or lasting pain.

Nothing in the wide world of exercise can compare to resistance training when it comes to creating the body you want. It can be performed anywhere . . . without any equipment. Resistance training exercise generally involves lifting weights, but can be accomplished by using either all or part of your body weight as a resistance, or moving your body against some externally imposed resistance, such as elastic resistance bands, free weights, or a strength-training machine.

If you are adamant about achieving peak physical fitness and having a great body, resistance training must be an essential part of your training regimen. That's because resistance training is the single best way to break down muscle tissue, which forces the body to adapt by adding more and bigger muscle cells during repair. Simply put, you tear down muscle during a workout, and your body builds it back up again. The best part is that building new muscle cells takes energy, in the form of calories. So you are not only getting bigger muscles, you're burning calories at an increased rate and diminishing body fat.

Resistance Training Benefits Your Entire Body

Men who put resistance or strength training on the back burner are missing a golden opportunity to reap maximum benefits. Studies have shown the importance of strength training in the prevention and rehabilitation of many chronic disease problems, such as physical dysfunction, obesity/low metabolism, weight control, osteoporosis, lower back pain, and heart disease.

In 2010, I was able to increase my own muscle mass by seven pounds through resistance training. This number is actually pretty staggering, because until very recently, the scientific community believed that men were destined to only lose muscle mass and strength as they age.

RESISTANCE TRAINING BURNS CALORIES

Resistance training improves both muscular strength and endurance and helps you not only prevent muscle loss that occurs with the aging process, but also creates new gains in muscle size and strength. After an intense workout, your body repairs the damaged muscle with a combination of sleep, rest, and nutrition, thus increasing your caloric needs over the next several days. Train hard often enough, and your body will be conditioned to constantly burn calories, day and night. And since all that repaired muscle is now bigger muscle—which takes more kilocalories to maintain—your basal metabolic rate increases. Basically, the more muscle you have, the more kilocalories you burn, even when you're asleep.

Aggressive resistance training is the first line of defense against sarcopenia. Although both aerobic and strength training are necessary for overall fitness, muscle and strength loss can be stopped and reversed only with resistance exercise.

As muscle mass decreases, resting metabolic rate (RMR), muscle strength, and activity levels also decrease. As our RMR declines, our calorie requirements also decline. Most people, however, don't reduce their caloric intake, and their body fat gradually increases each year. The increased body fat—and the accompanying increase in abdominal obesity and hidden visceral fat—promotes many serious disease states, including insulin resistance and dyslipidemia (high cholesterol, low HDL, high triglycerides, and high LDL), which damages blood vessels and causes heart disease and heart attack, the number-one killer of American men.

Strength training also helps maintain and even increase bone density, further reducing the risk of fractures. In fact, high-intensity strength training is the only type of exercise that will prevent and actually treat osteoporosis and other degenerative bone diseases.

Here is a quick list of other health issues that strength training improves:

- **Mitochondrial transformation:** As you crank out your reps and sets, you are transforming old, defective, damaged, and mutated mitochondria that I described in Chapter 4 into new, healthy, vibrant, wild-type mitochondria capable of producing huge quantities of ATP, which not only will energize you, but also will make you stronger and feel younger.

- **Improved cognitive and physical function:** The combination of strength training, cardiovascular training, and exercises that involve quick controlled moves (like martial arts) work synergistically as a protective factor for cognitive decline and dementia.

- **Gain in insulin sensitivity and reduced Metabolic Syndrome:** Regular resistance training plays a key role in the prevention of the accumulation of abdominal fat and the subsequent development of insulin resistance, the major cause of type 2 diabetes and heart disease.

- **Improved posture, balance, and core strength:** Balance and coordination are also improved with weight lifting by increasing strength, muscle size, muscle endurance, and joint range of motion, thereby reducing your chance of falling, fractures, and debilitation.

- **Improved sexual function:** Muscle mass and strength are important for all types of physical activity, including sex. You need to have a lean, fit, strong, flexible body to guarantee outstanding sexual performance.

Strength Training Alleviates Back Pain

I have had to deal with back pain, as have literally hundreds of my patients. Lower back pain affects 90 percent of all American men at some point, and is the fifth-most-common reason for all physician visits. Eighty-five percent of all back pain is localized to the lower back. Most men do recover from episodes of lower back pain, but a small percentage don't and go on to develop chronic problems, especially if they resume full activities too quickly and reinjure the same area.

There are two kinds of back pain: acute and chronic. Acute pain usually does not last longer than three months and is best treated by your doctor with analgesics (pain medicines) and a continuation of normal activities as tolerated. An exercise program can be resumed gradually but must be performed very carefully to avoid aggravating the injury.

Chronic low back pain (pain that persists longer than three months) must be evaluated by a physician to exclude serious underlying diseases, such as cancer, osteoporosis, rheumatologic disease (a very serious form of arthritis), infection, or a herniated disc. Most cases of chronic low back pain (85 to 90 percent) are caused by simple strains and sprains of muscles, ligaments, or tendons located in the lumbosacral area.

While all forms of exercise have been shown to benefit people with chronic low back pain, an intense, integrated approach like the Life Plan has been proven to be the most effective. This strategy not only improves endurance and activity tolerance but also increases the strength and flexibility of your back muscles. In addition, it promotes weight loss (obesity is a major cause of acute and chronic back pain) and provides beneficial psychological effects.

In a study published last year in the *Archives of Physical Medicine and Rehabilitation*, Dr. B. W. Nelson and colleagues set out to determine if back-pain patients recommended for spinal surgery could avoid their surgery through an aggressive strengthening program. After following a 10-week intensive back-strengthening regimen, 57 of the 60 patients no longer required surgery and were virtually pain free. There are well over 100 other studies that have shown that cardiovascular and strength-training exercises can alleviate chronic back pain by strengthening and increasing the flexibility of back muscles.

It is critically important to see your doctor before you start a resistance training program, especially if you suffer frequently from back pain. Once you get the green light from your doctor, focus on exercises that strengthen the muscles that support your back, which include the abdominal and low back muscles. Be sure to conduct your exercises in a slow and controlled manner, and always use perfect form with each exercise.

Resistance Training Enhances The Life Plan

It may not be the body fat you see, but the fat you don't that is doing you the greatest harm. Visceral fat lurks under the abdominal muscle inside your abdominal cavity and can snake its way around internal organs. Studies show the more visceral fat you have, the more at risk you are of developing Metabolic Syndrome, diabetes, hypertension, cardiovascular disease, some cancers, and Alzheimer's.

In fact, a 2006 study published in the online edition of *Obesity* compared visceral, subcu-

"Being an owner of a general contracting firm and development company, I am working outside on projects almost all year. At 48 years and quickly approaching the age when my father had his first heart attack (50), with open-heart surgery at 52, I knew that I did not want to relive his experience.

"I've been told that I am the duplicate of my father's weight, height, and even his high cholesterol levels. At 238 pounds and six-two, I worked out three to four days per week, and I thought I was in pretty good shape. I knew I needed to start seeing a doctor on a yearly basis. I wanted one who understood how to train, eat properly, and rest.

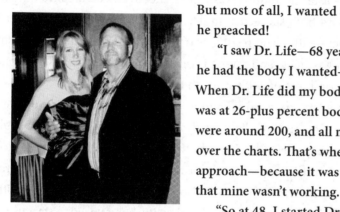

But most of all, I wanted a doctor who practiced what he preached!

"I saw Dr. Life—68 years young at that time, and he had the body I wanted—lean, toned, and muscular! When Dr. Life did my body analysis, I was shocked. I was at 26-plus percent body fat, my cholesterol levels were around 200, and all my other levels were all over the charts. That's when I decided to try Dr. Life's approach—because it was clear that mine wasn't working.

"So at 48, I started Dr. Life's program. I steadily improved over time, dropping body fat and adding muscle mass. It is nice going to the doctor's office and having him tell you you're doing well instead of you're overweight and heading for a heart attack. I follow Dr. Life's instructions to the letter, even bagging my vitamins for long trips.

"This year at my annual body analysis, my body fat is 9.2 percent, and since I've started, I have gained 26 pounds of muscle mass. I weigh 201 pounds and feel great. More than ever, I now enjoy working out five to six days per week and golf as often as two to three times per week—all without any pain.

"THANK YOU, DR. LIFE—for helping me achieve the fitness level that will take me long into my golden years."

taneous, and liver fat levels in Texas men and found that "visceral fat alone independently predicted risk of mortality after adjustment for the other fat measures." However, we do know that men who exercise tended to lose more visceral fat than those who merely dieted to lose weight.

But what type of exercise was best? To find out which is better at fighting fat—resistance or aerobic training—exercise physiologists at the University of Alabama's Department of Human Studies divided 97 subjects into three groups: aerobic training, resistance training, and no exercise. Participants followed a restricted-calorie diet and lost an average of 24 pounds each. Afterward, the two exercise groups were instructed to continue their exercise regimen (40 minutes, two times a week) for a year.

The findings revealed that resistance training was just as effective as aerobic training in preventing the regaining of fat, and both succeeded in decreasing harmful visceral fat. Yet I see many men at the gym who focus entirely on resistance training, and their bellies still seem distended. My experience with my patients and myself is that if you tend to store fat in your abdomen you must do cardio in combination with strength training to get rid of it.

Aerobic exercise and resistance training work hand in hand to prevent, reduce, or even reverse heart disease by preventing/controlling diabetes, dyslipidemia (high cholesterol, high triglycerides, and low HDL), and hypertension. They do this through all the complex biochemical and physiological processes that are initiated during these exercises and for several hours after they are completed. Both forms of exercise also strengthen the heart. Men with healthy hearts—no matter what their age—and most with unhealthy hearts need to start using resistance training along with their aerobic training as an important part of their heart-disease prevention and/or treatment program.

The "How" of Resistance Training

The components of a good resistance training program include strengthening every muscle group in your body: legs, arms, back, shoulders, and core. Most people think the core is synonymous with abdominal muscles. The "core" actually consists of many different muscles that stabilize the spine and pelvis and run the entire length of the torso. These muscles provide a solid foundation for movement in the extremities.

Training of all these muscle groups is done by completing various exercises, at a particular frequency (how many times you repeat the same movement), duration (how long you hold a particular pose), and intensity (how much weight you are working with).

You will need to incorporate resistance training into your exercise program three to four days per week to achieve the best results for your body.

I suggest that you make the following rules your mantra:

- Make resistance training a key component of your exercise program. My exercise regimen starts with resistance training five days a week.

- Train as if your life depends on it—because it does. If I hadn't started training 13 years ago for the Body-*for*-LIFE contest and added the Cenegenics program to my regimen five years later, I wouldn't be alive today. It's really that simple.

- Train like a 30-year-old—unless, of course, you are 30, then train as if you are 20. Always set the bar higher. Never stay in your comfort zone.

- Achieve new heights in the "no pain no gain" attitude.

- You must achieve muscle soreness (good pain) after each training session. Good pain is soreness that is on both sides of your body, not sharp or extreme, just enough to let you know that you worked your muscles just right. It's a great feeling.

SORE MUSCLES

1. It's normal to have some muscle pain after a good workout. In fact, this is usually a good indication that you trained your muscles properly. Occasionally, however, this pain can be excessive and may even interfere with your training program. Ibuprofen, or another nonsteroidal anti-inflammatory drug, is frequently used to alleviate this kind of pain, but these medications can interfere with your muscle repair and growth processes. I never take them for this kind of muscle discomfort. Instead, I take my vitamins.

2. Scientists believe the muscle pain associated with intense exercise is caused, in part, by the excessive production of free radicals (very active molecules) during exercise. Free radicals help repair the microscopic tears and inflammation we want to produce in our muscle tissue when we train hard, and they actually promote increases in strength and growth. Excessive amounts of these molecules, however, can actually do more harm than good and interfere with muscle healing.

3. We have known for some time now that antioxidant supplements, including vitamin E, vitamin C, and selenium, help neutralize free-radical activity. They may help prevent the excessive muscle damage from free radicals that intense exercise can cause. So train hard, take your antioxidants, eat healthy, and enjoy the "good" pain you get in your muscles after a great workout.

Strengthening the Whole Body

- -

On the Life Plan I recommend doing a total body workout three to four days a week. It is very important to train your whole body in a way that stresses every muscle over the course of the week. By doing so, you will be gaining the benefit of burning more calories than you would by just doing one muscle group per day. Training the whole body during a workout, particularly a circuit workout, causes the heart to work harder to pump blood and oxygen to the muscles that are performing the work. This results in a higher heart rate, which equates to a higher caloric expenditure.

DETERMINE YOUR 1-REP MAX

A phrase you'll hear often in this chapter is "your 1-rep max." In short, it's the heaviest weight you can lift for one rep of a particular exercise. To determine your 1-rep max, use the calculators on my website (www.drlife.com). All you have to do is enter the amount of weight that you lifted and the number of reps you were able to perform, and the calculator will estimate your 1-rep max. Choose a weight with which you can do no more than 10 reps to determine your 1-rep max.

The danger of not training the whole body in a balanced way is that you set yourself up for muscle imbalances, postural distortions, and interference with reciprocal inhibition (when muscles on the opposite sides of a joint contract at the same time, producing muscle tears), causing undue stress on the joints and soft tissues of your body. All that means just one thing: injury. You do not want to injure yourself. Injuries can set you back months and in some cases, years. Avoid injuries at all costs. Move slowly through your exercise journey. It's meant for a lifetime, not 12 weeks.

Getting Strength Training Started

- -

Whether you begin with the Basic Health program or jump into a higher level, if you already have experience with resistance training, your workout will contain the same core components:

- Warmup

- Exercise

- Cool-down

Before you begin your resistance training it is important to prepare your body mentally and physically to perform exercise. You should treat warming up as seriously as the workout itself. A proper warmup will not only get you physically and mentally ready to work out, but it also improves your performance significantly. When your muscles are warmed up they will contract more forcefully and relax more quickly, which decreases the risk of overstretching or overstressing your muscle.

A general warmup could be walking on the treadmill, riding a stationary or street bike, or running for three to five minutes, followed by a couple of light sets of your first strength-training exercise. Or you could just do a specific warmup for a particular exercise. For example, before working out on the bench press, you could do two lighter sets with just the bar before performing your actual "working" sets. Or, if you plan to perform a bench press with 75 percent of your 1-rep max, your warmup can be a few sets with 30 to 40 percent of your 1-rep max. This will prepare your body to perform more efficiently at a higher intensity.

The Life Plan Workout is designed with a warmup built in. If you follow the workout as it is designed in Chapter 8, you will not need to do an additional warmup. However, if you want to add an additional resistance training workout to your week, then you must warm up first.

PREVENTING LEG CRAMPS

Near the end of a hard set of hamstring curls, you may feel a cramp starting to come on and find that you have to stop the set. These cramps are usually a result of poor conditioning, sluggish blood flow to the muscles, and poor flexibility. Flexibility is a very important aspect of our total conditioning, but most of us choose to ignore it. Tight muscles get much less blood circulating through them than relaxed muscles. In a flexible person, blood moves freely and unimpeded through the exercising muscles, flushing out lactic acid and providing vital oxygen to muscle cells. It is this lack of oxygen combined with high levels of lactic acid that can cause pain and cramping.

If you include stretching exercises as an integral part of your overall conditioning program, you can prevent cramping and delay the development of fatigue. Stretching also helps avoid injury and improves overall performance. Also, be sure you're conducting your exercises through the full range of motion. This will ensure a good stretch on the eccentric (negative) portion of the movement.

If your hamstrings cramp up, as mine used to, just massage the muscle, stretch it out, and get back to work. As your strength, conditioning, and flexibility improve, these cramps will soon become a thing of the past.

Performing the Resistance Exercise

The actual exercise is measured in repetitions and sets. A repetition is one complete movement of a particular exercise. There are three phases of a repetition:

1. Eccentric contraction—when you are resisting the pull of gravity by not allowing the weight to fall on your chest.

2. Isometric contraction of the muscle—when the muscle is static and the opposing force (the weight) is not being moved at all.

3. Concentric contraction—the positive portion of the lift where the muscle shortens to exert force against the weight (for example, when you push the barbell up—against gravity).

The speed—or tempo—at which you perform a repetition is determined by your fitness goals. If you have not been working out consistently in the past, it's important to increase your muscular endurance before you focus solely on developing increased strength. The Basic Health Workout will focus on endurance, while the two remaining levels will help you achieve both.

For example, if your goal is increased strength, the tempo should be slower to allow the muscle and ligaments enough time under tension to increase in size. A good tempo for this would be 4-2-2, that is, a 4-second count during the eccentric portion, a 2-second count during the isometric portion, and a 2-second count during the concentric portion. For strength gain, a 2-2-2 tempo would be more appropriate.

The Set

A number of repetitions performed one after another make up a set. If you are starting at the Basic Health Workout, you will start with endurance training, which has a higher rep range and fewer sets. This helps build muscular endurance and enables the nervous system to learn the correct movements and how to recruit the right muscles during each particular exercise, decreasing the risk of injury.

The general rule is it takes 500 reps of a particular exercise to train your body to perform it correctly. You shouldn't train to muscle failure until your body has reached the point of total comfort with the exercise. Once you've got the form down pat, and your nervous system, joints, and muscle stabilizers are strong enough to keep the weight steady, you can then go to muscle failure. At that point, you can also branch out into other types of training if desired, such as strength training, where the optimal rep range is 6 to 8 repetitions and 3 to 4 sets.

The Rest Period

Between sets, you should take a break. In endurance training, the rest period between sets is usually 30 to 60 seconds; in strength training, 2 to 3 minutes.

Intensity

Intensity refers to the amount of force you should use—that is, how heavy the weight should be. Endurance training uses an intensity of 50 to 70 percent of your 1-rep max (again, each repetition should be at a weight equal to 50 to 70 percent of the maximum amount of weight you can lift on that particular exercise if you do it only one time). Strength training uses 75 to 85 percent of 1-rep max.

The Cool-Down Period

Each session should end with a cool-down period, such as walking/running on the treadmill or getting on the stair stepper for five minutes at about 45 to 50 percent of your target heart rate to bring your body back to a resting state. Stretching is an excellent way to cool down. The Life Plan Workout is designed with a cool-down built in. If you follow the workout as it is designed in Chapter 8, you will not need to do an additional cool-down. However, if you want to add an additional resistance training workout to your week, then you must add stretching when you are done.

TRAINING WITH A PARTNER

We tend to perform better when we have someone there to push us. It always helps to have a workout partner, either a friend or a trainer, someone there to motivate you to push yourself a little bit harder than you would by yourself. And, for many resistance training exercises, it's just not safe to get to muscle failure without someone there to spot you—someone who knows what he or she is doing.

The Basic Health Resistance Workout

If you are just beginning a resistance training program, it is wise to get your body acclimated by slowly easing into the workout. Start small, finding the exercises that you enjoy and that you will look forward to performing regularly.

There are some simple rules and guidelines you need to follow to maximize your success. First, start with 2 to 3 sets per exercise, 15 to 25 repetitions, and 45- to 90-second rest periods. Each rep should be performed at a slow pace of around 6 seconds.

For example, each of the suggested exercises will look like this: *Barbell Bench Press—100 lbs, 2 to 3 sets of 15 to 25 repetitions, 45- to 90-second rest after each.*

The purpose of the higher repetitions and short rest periods is to build your muscular endurance as well as increase the integrity of the joints and connective tissues. Beginners do not possess high levels of neuromuscular control, so it's important to perform your sets with lighter weights to help increase your ability to stabilize the weights. It is important not to rush the speed of the repetitions. Perform all repetitions at a 3-2-1 tempo (3 seconds eccentric, 2 seconds isometric, 1 second concentric).

A full-body routine is more advantageous during this phase, as the goal is not to increase muscle size and strength but to train your nervous system to interact with your muscular system. You should continue with this phase for four to six weeks.

The following is a sample workout. It is also suitable to perform this routine in a circuit fashion three days a week. Perform one set of each exercise without a break, and then repeat until you have completed three sets of each exercise. Performing a circuit will increase your heart rate and allow you to burn more calories. Just be sure to have at least one day between workouts for recovery. If there is still muscle soreness with one day of rest, wait an extra day to repeat the workout.

1. Warmup: 5–10 minutes

2. The circuit

CHEST				
Incline DB press	2–3 sets	25 reps	45–90 sec rest	Tempo 3-2-1
BACK				
Seated row	2–3 sets	25 reps	45–90 sec rest	Tempo 3-2-1

Overhead dumbbell press	2–3 sets	25 reps	45–90 sec rest	Tempo 3-2-1
LEGS				
Leg press	2–3 sets	25 reps	45–90 sec rest	Tempo 3-2-1

3. Cool-down stretching: 5–10 minutes

The Fitness Resistance Training Workout

When you feel comfortable at the gym and have completed the Basic Health Workout, you are ready to increase your intensity. During this next phase we will focus more on increasing lean muscle and decreasing body fat percentage. The percentage of your 1-rep max is greater in this phase in order to place enough stress on the muscle tissues to break them down, which forces your body to increase the size of the muscles to adapt to the increased load. If you don't have a workout partner by now, you may want to seriously look into getting one: It is difficult and dangerous to perform workouts with heavier weights without a spotter.

The protocol for this phase is 3 to 4 sets, 6 to 12 repetitions, and 75 to 85 percent of your 1-rep max, tempo 4-2-1 (4 seconds eccentric, 2 seconds isometric, 1 second concentric), with 30- to 60-second rest periods.

Example: If your lateral pull-downs 1-rep max was 100 pounds, you would do: *Lateral pull-downs—75 to 85 lbs, 3 to 5 sets, 8 to 12 reps, 30- to 60-second rest period between sets.*

During this phase a split routine is recommended: On one day you will work on your chest/shoulders/triceps, then the next workout you will concentrate on back/biceps/legs. This phase should be performed four days a week, alternating between workouts twice a week, for at least four weeks.

Day One

1. Warmup: 5–10 minutes

2. Day One routine

   CHEST

a) Incline press b) Machine fly	3–5 sets each exercise	8–12 reps per set	75–85% of max	4-2-1 tempo	60–90 sec rest after each set

   SHOULDERS

a) EZ curl bar upright row b) Dumbbell lateral raise	3–5 sets each exercise	8–12 reps per set	75–85% of max	4-2-1 tempo	60–90 sec rest after each set

   TRICEPS

a) Lying overhead extension b) Kick backs	3–5 sets each exercise	8–12 reps per set	75–85% of max	4-2-1 tempo	60–90 sec rest after each set

3. Cool-down/stretching: 5–10 minutes

Day Two

1. Warmup: 5–10 minutes

2. Day Two routine

   BACK

a) Lat pull-down b) Dumbbell row	3–5 sets each exercise	8–12 reps per set	75–85% of max	4-2-1 tempo	60–90 sec rest after each set

   BICEPS

a) Cable curl b) Dumbbell curl	3–5 sets each exercise	8–12 reps per set	75–85% of max	4-2-1 tempo	60–90 sec rest after each set

   LEGS

a) Barbell lunges b) Straight leg dead lift	3–5 sets each exercise	8–12 reps per set	75–85% of max	4-2-1 tempo	60–90 sec rest after each set

3. Cool-down/stretching: 5–10 minutes

The High-Performance Resistance Training Workout

Strength and power are the focal point for this phase. Once you have completed six weeks of fitness resistance training you should be ready to move to this stage. There are no shortcuts, and by jumping into this phase of training prematurely you will interfere with muscle growth and strength gains: If your muscles aren't really ready you will experience soft-tissue/joint injuries. The two previous levels are designed to prepare your body to perform at max level intensity with higher weight loads.

You will now increase your workload to an even higher percentage of your 1-rep max. The increase of the workload and the speed at which the repetitions are performed make this workout advanced. The two exercises per body part should be completed with no break in between, then you should take the rest period allotted. During this phase the protocol is 4 to 6 sets, 5 reps, 85 to 100 percent of max with 3 to 5 minutes rest. There is no specified tempo during this phase of training. A spotter is definitely required.

You will complete a more isolated split routine. This phase should be performed four days a week, alternating between workouts twice a week, for at least four weeks.

Example: If your bench press 1-rep max is 100 pounds you would perform: *Bench Press— 85 to 100 lbs, 5 reps, 4 to 6 sets, 3- to 5-min rest periods, 3-2-1 tempo.*

Day One

1. Warmup: 5–10 minutes

2. Day One routine

   BACK

a) Barbell row	4–6 sets	5 reps	85–100%	Tempo fast as can be controlled	Complete both exercises then rest 3–5 min
b) Crunch to jump pull-up					

   CHEST

a) Bench press	4–6 sets	5 reps	85–100%	Tempo fast as can be controlled	Complete both exercises then rest 3–5 min
b) Power pushups					

3. Cool-down/stretching: 5–10 minutes

Day Two

1. Warmup: 5–10 minutes

2. Day Two routine

LEGS

a) Barbell squat	4–6 sets	5 reps	85–100%	Tempo fast as can be controlled	Complete both exercises then rest 3–5 min
b) Squat jump knee tuck					

BICEPS

a) Squat to curl	4–6 sets	5 reps	85–100%	Tempo fast as can be controlled	Complete both exercises then rest 3–5 min
b) Preacher curl					

3. Cool-down/stretching: 5–10 minutes

Day Three

1. Warmup: 5–10 minutes

2. Day Three routine

SHOULDERS

a) Power push press	4–6 sets	5 reps	85–100%	Tempo fast as can be controlled	Complete both exercises then rest 3–5 min
b) EZ curl bar upright row					

TRICEPS

a) Dips	4–6 sets	5 reps	85–100%	Tempo fast as can be controlled	Complete both exercises then rest 3–5 min
b) Pushdowns					

3. Cool-down/stretching: 5–10 minutes

How to Keep Training When You're on the Road

Maintaining a training routine at a gym is relatively easy. You need to *just do it!* Pick the time of day that works best for you and don't miss it—ever. When the thought of not going to the gym enters your head, quickly visualize the lean, fit, muscular body you want and focus on that. Work with a trainer or training partner who will give you a hard time if you are a no-show. And when you are working out, concentrate on your form for each exercise. Check out your body in the mirrors and focus on the muscle group you are exercising. Keep a journal of your performance, photos, weight, percentage of body fat, grams of muscle tissue, and waist, biceps, and chest measurements.

If you train at home, make sure you have plenty of mirrors to keep track of your progress. They are really important. When you finish the last rep you can do of a set . . . do another one. When you are on the road, it's much harder to stay on track. You need to think ahead. Make sure there is a good gym in the vicinity where you will be staying before you leave. Take exercise bands with you and a jump rope so you can work out in your hotel room. Do chair dips, pushups with your feet on the floor, on a chair, and on the dresser. Do front rising kicks and air punches in your room—250 of each, 2 to 3 sets. Walk/run outside. Be creative and you will be amazed at what a great workout you can get when you are traveling. And by all means, continue to eat clean.

Resistance Training Exercises

Following are a group of exercises. Some of them are listed in each of the individual workouts. Others are included for you to change up your program. It's important to vary your exercises as you progress through the levels of training. Don't stay with one exercise for more than three weeks. Feel free to change any time you want. If you aren't really excited by a particular exercise, switch to another. If you are not an advanced resistance trainer I would advise holding off on the advanced exercises until you or your trainer believe you are ready for them.

All of these exercises can be used in any of the three phases of training, with the exception of exercises that require an explosive action (e.g., power pushups or squat jumps). These exercises are interchangeable because each phase of training will manipulate several variables (tempo, rest period, percentage of max, etc.) that will provide a different effect while utilizing the same exercise. Explosive exercises should be used where a tempo of 1-1-1 is recommended. Be sure to follow the outlined protocol for each phase of workouts for maximum benefits.

BENCH PRESS

Benefits: This exercise primarily strengthens the chest.

To start: Lie on a flat bench. Keep your feet flat and draw your navel inward. With your arms fully extended, grasp the barbell a little farther than shoulder width apart.

1. With the arms extended, lift the bar off the bench.

2. In a controlled manner lower the bar toward your chest until the upper part of your arm (triceps) is parallel with the floor, forming a 90-degree angle.

3. Press the bar upward using your pectoral muscles. Straighten your arms fully, stopping just before you lock out the elbows.

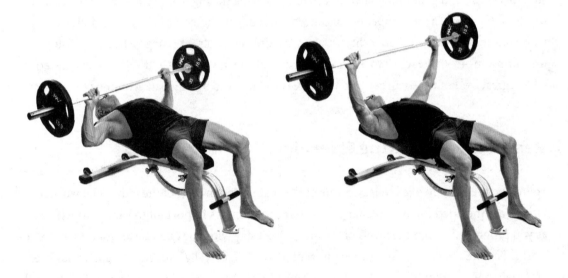

DUMBBELL CHEST PRESS

Benefits: This exercise shapes and strengthens your chest.

To start: Lie on your back on a flat bench. Hold a dumbbell in each hand on both sides of your chest. Pull your navel inward.

1. Lifting both weights at the same pace, push them straight up until your arms are fully extended.

2. Hold them there for 1 second, and then return to the starting position.

3. When lowering the dumbbells stop when the upper arm (triceps) is parallel to the floor.

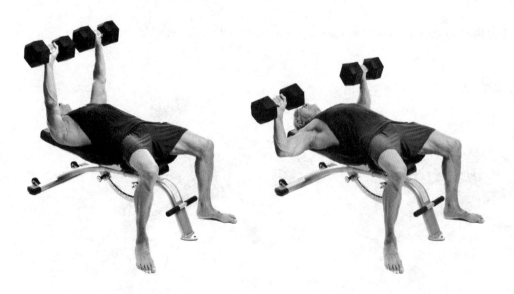

DUMBBELL FLY

Benefits: This exercise shapes and strengthens your chest.

To start: Lie down on an exercise bench with your feet flat on the floor. Draw your navel inward. Grab a pair of dumbbells with palms facing each other.

1. Extend your arms above your chest, elbows slightly bent. Pinch your shoulder blades against the pad.

2. Lower your arms out to your sides to about shoulder level.

3. Begin to contract your chest muscles to bring your arms together, forming an arc with your arms.

NOTE: For the at-home workout, lie over a physio ball to do this exercise.

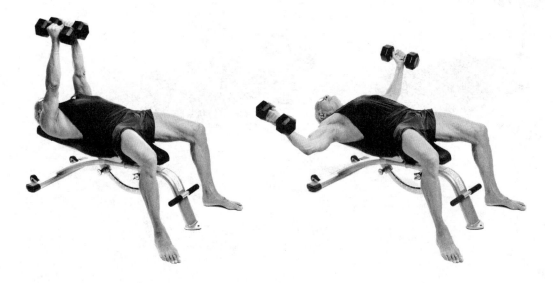

MACHINE PRESS

Benefits: This exercise shapes and strengthens your chest.

To start: Sit on the seated press machine, with your back firmly against the pad, your feet flat on the floor. Draw your navel inward. Adjust the seat so that machine handles are in line with your upper chest. Grasp the handles with a palms-down grip.

1. Push against the machine handles and extend your arm in front of you, contracting your chest muscles.

2. Slowly lower the handles back to the starting position without letting the weight stack touch. Stop when your arms form a 90-degree angle.

INCLINE DUMBBELL PRESS

Benefits: This exercise shapes and strengthens your chest.

To start: Lie on an incline bench set at approximately a 30- to 45-degree angle. Keep your feet flat on the floor and draw your navel inward. Grab a pair of dumbbells, with a palms-down grip.

1. Extend your arms fully so the dumbbells are directly above your chest almost touching each other. Pinch your shoulder blades against the pad.

2. Slowly lower the dumbbell to shoulder level. Your elbows should form a 90-degree angle.

3. Press the dumbbell upward, using your pectoral muscle. Straighten your arms fully and squeeze at the top.

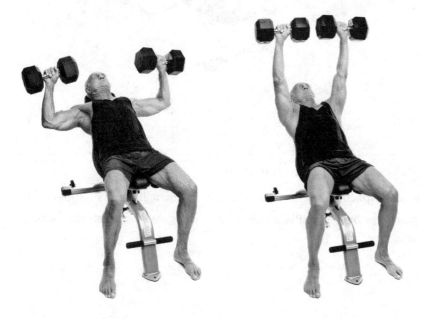

DECLINE DUMBBELL PRESS

Benefits: This exercise shapes and strengthens your chest.

To start: Lie on a decline bench. Draw your navel inward. Grab a pair of dumbbells, with a palms-down grip. You may need a spotter to hand you the dumbbells.

1. Extend your arms fully so the dumbbells are directly above your chest almost touching each other. Pinch your shoulder blades against the pad.

2. Slowly lower the dumbbell to shoulder level. Your elbows should form a 90-degree angle.

3. Press the dumbbell upward, using your pectoral muscle. Straighten your arms fully and squeeze at the top.

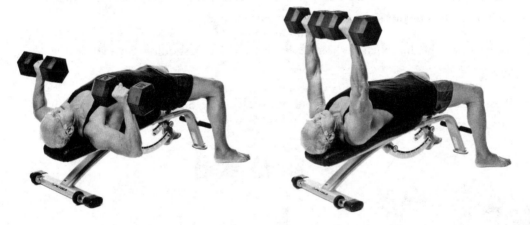

MACHINE FLY

Benefits: This exercise shapes and strengthens your chest.

To start: Adjust the seat of the machine so that your arms are in line with your shoulders. Sit with your torso erect against the back pad. Place your forearms against the resistance pads. Draw your navel inward.

1. Push the resistance pads toward each other and contract your chest muscles hard at the top of the movement.

2. Slowly return your arms to start until your elbows are in line with your shoulders.

NOTE: Make sure your shoulders maintain full contact with the back pad.

PUSHUPS

Benefits: This exercise shapes and strengthens your chest.

To start: Place your hands on the floor, slightly wider than shoulder width apart, and extend your legs behind you, your toes on the floor.

1. Lower your body by bending your elbows until your upper-arm bicep is parallel to the floor.

2. Press up until your arms are straight. Stop before you lock your elbows. Return to the starting position.

VARIATION: If standard pushups are too difficult, place your hands on a low bench.

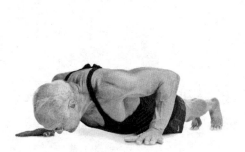 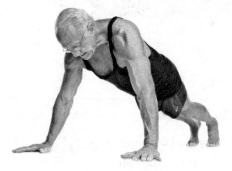

ADVANCED POWER PUSHUP

Benefits: This exercise shapes and strengthens your chest as well as develops explosive power—a fast burst of maximum effort.

To start: Place your hands on the floor, slightly wider than shoulder width apart, and extend your legs behind you, your toes on the floor.

1. Complete a standard pushup with the following timing: slow and controlled on the way down.

2. Push up as fast as you can, catching a bit of air at the top.

3. Repeat for the prescribed number of reps.

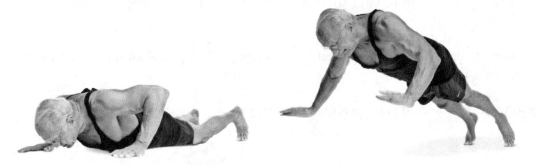

PUSHUP CLAP

Benefits: This exercise shapes and strengthens your chest as well as develops explosive power.

To start: Place your hands on the floor, slightly wider than shoulder width apart, and extend your legs behind you, your toes on the floor.

1. Complete a standard pushup with the following timing: slow and controlled on the way down.

2. Push up as fast as you can, catching a bit of air at the top.

3. Clap your hands together between pushups.

4. Repeat for the prescribed number of reps.

Back

LAT PULL-DOWN

Benefits: This exercise shapes and strengthens your upper back.

To start: Sit at the lateral pull-down machine. Adjust the knee pads so that they fit snugly over your thighs. Place your feet flat on the floor. Draw your navel inward. Keep your torso erect. Grasp the bar with your palms facing away from your body.

1. Draw your shoulder blades together and pull the bar down toward your chest, just past your chin.

2. Hold this position for 2 seconds.

3. Slowly straighten your arms, bringing the bar overhead.

SEATED ROW

Benefits: This exercise strengthens and shapes your back.

To start: Sit down on seated-row bench machine. Draw your navel inward. Keep your back straight. Place your feet on the platform with your legs slightly bent. Choose a handle that has a double neutral grip (palms facing inward) and attach to the lower pulley cable.

1. Hold the handles and pull them toward your midsection.

2. Pull your shoulder blades together and contract your back muscles.

3. Extend your arms in front of you. Stop before your shoulder blades roll forward.

NOTE: Be sure to keep your torso erect.

BENT-OVER DUMBBELL ROW

Benefits: This exercise strengthens and shapes your back and hamstrings.

To start: Stand with your feet shoulder width apart or slightly narrower with a slight bend in your knees, holding a dumbbell in each hand.

1. Hinge yourself at the hips without losing the natural curve in your back. Your back should be almost parallel to the floor.

2. Bring the weights toward your chest by bending your elbows and squeezing your shoulder blades together without shrugging your shoulders. Return to the starting position.

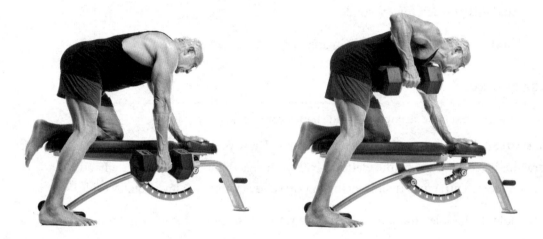

Benefits: This exercise strengthens the muscles in the upper back.

To start: Grab the overhead bar with your palms facing away from your body slightly wider than shoulder width apart. Extend your arms and relax your shoulders to fully stretch your back. Draw your navel inward.

1. Pull yourself up until your chin is even with the bar.

2. Contract your back at the top of the movement.

3. Slowly lower to the starting position.

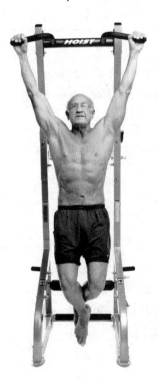
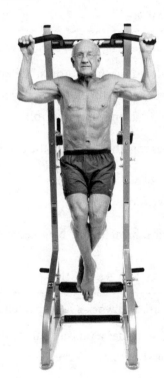

BACK EXTENSION

Benefits: This exercise will strengthen the low back, gluteus, and hamstrings.

To start: Position your body on the machine with your legs about hip width apart. Place your hands on your chest and draw your navel inward. Keep knees slightly bent.

1. In a controlled manner lean forward at the waist.

2. When your body is at about a 45-degree angle, stop.

3. Return to the starting position by contracting the gluteus, hamstrings, and lower back.

REVERSE GRIP PULL-DOWN

Benefits: This exercise shapes and strengthens your upper back.

To start: Sit at the lateral pull-down machine. Adjust the knee pads so that they fit snugly over your thighs. Place your feet flat on the floor. Draw your navel inward. Keep your torso erect. Grasp the bar with a palms-facing-inward grip.

1. Draw your shoulder blades together and pull the bar down toward your chest, just past your chin.

2. Hold this position for 2 seconds.

3. Slowly straighten your arms, bringing the bar overhead.

ADVANCED CRUNCH TO JUMP PULL-UP

Benefits: This total-body exercise will work a large percentage of your back and legs.

To start: Place a mat on the floor, under a pull-up bar. Lie flat on your back, with bottom of feet flat on the floor. Your arms should be overhead.

1. Begin by swinging your arms from overhead toward your feet.

2. Allow the momentum of the arm swing to carry your body into a full sit-up.

3. Allow the momentum of the sit-up, combined with the strength of your legs, to get you up off the floor.

4. As soon as your body is upright, jump up to grasp the pull-up bars.

5. Pull your body up until your chin is over the bar.

6. Lower your body off the bar onto your feet.

7. Sit back on the floor.

8. Once you are seated, lie back on the floor in your original starting position.

BARBELL ROW

Benefits: Works the middle part of back, particularly the rhomboids and rear delts.

To start: Stand upright, holding a barbell with palms facing inward. Keep your back straight and bend forward at the waist. Draw your navel inward. Keep your knees slightly bent. Extend your arms straight down.

1. Pull the barbell toward your chest. Concentrate on pulling with your back muscles.

2. Raise your elbows as high as possible.

3. Slowly lower your arms, returning to the starting position.

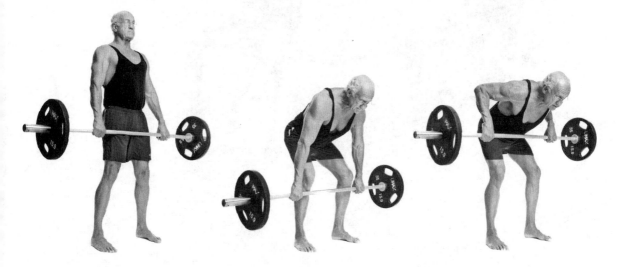

OVERHEAD DUMBBELL PRESS

Benefits: This exercise shapes and strengthens the front of your shoulders.

To start: Sitting on the end of a bench, or on a seated bench apparatus, bring two dumbbells to shoulder height.

1. Press the weights directly overhead until your arms are fully extended.

2. Return to the starting position. Upper arm (triceps) should remain parallel to the floor.

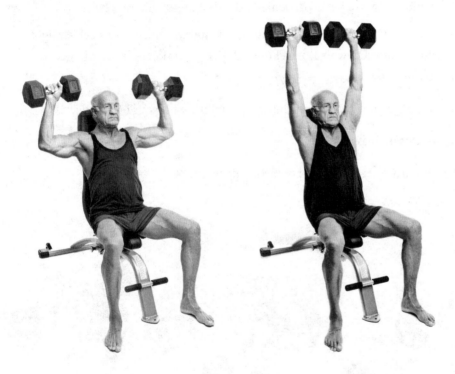

STANDING DUMBBELL SHOULDER PRESS

Benefits: This exercise shapes and strengthens the front of your shoulders.

To start: Stand with your feet shoulder width apart. Hold a dumbbell in each hand and lift them until upper arms/triceps are parallel to the floor.

1. Press the weights directly overhead until your arms are fully extended.

2. Return to the starting position. Upper arm (triceps) should remain parallel to the floor.

3. Repeat for prescribed number of repetitions.

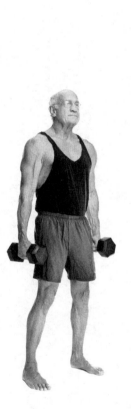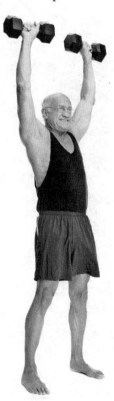

DUMBBELL LATERAL RAISE

Benefits: This exercise shapes and strengthens the sides of your shoulders.

To start: Stand erect with your feet closer than shoulder width apart. Draw your navel inward. Grab a pair of 5-pound dumbbells with a palm-down grip.

1. Extend your arms out to your sides to shoulder level. Keep your elbows slightly bent. Hold for 2 seconds.

2. Slowly lower to the starting position.

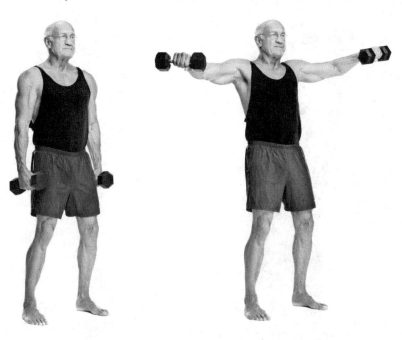

DUMBBELL FRONT RAISE

Benefits: This exercise shapes and strengthens your shoulders.

To start: Stand erect with your feet shoulder width apart. Draw your navel inward. Grab a pair of 5- or 10-pound dumbbells with a palms-down grip. Extend your arms straight down and in front of your thighs.

1. Raise your arms out in front of you to about shoulder level. Keep your elbows slightly bent.

2. Slowly lower the dumbbells back to the starting position.

EZ CURL BAR UPRIGHT ROW

Benefits: This exercise will shape and strengthen the sides of your shoulders and upper part of your back.

To start: Stand with your torso erect. Draw your navel inward. Grab a bar with both hands, using a palms-down grip. Rest your arms in front of your thighs. Your hands should be slightly closer than shoulder width apart.

1. Pull the bar straight up, using strength in your elbows, not your hands.

2. Raise your arms until they are a little above your chest level. Keep the barbell a few inches in front of your body.

3. Slowly return to the starting position.

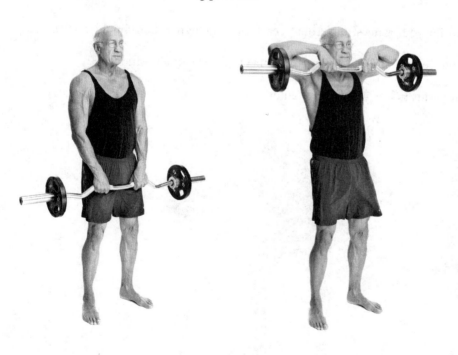

MACHINE REAR FLY

Benefits: This exercise shapes and strengthens the back of your shoulders and upper back.

To start: Sit facing the rear deltoid machine, placing your feet firmly on the floor. Grab the machine handles and draw your navel inward.

1. Begin by pulling on the machine handles and extend your arms to your sides.

2. Contract your shoulder and back muscles.

3. Slowly return to the starting position.

DUMBBELL BENT-OVER REAR FLY

Benefits: This exercise shapes and strengthens the rear part of your shoulders and upper back.

To start: Stand erect. Grab a pair of dumbbells with your palms facing each other. Bend at the waist, keeping your back straight and perpendicular to the floor. Draw your navel inward. Keep your knees slightly bent. There should be a slight arch in your lower back. Extend your arms and look forward.

1. Begin by raising your arms straight out to each side, no higher than shoulder level.

2. Contract your rear shoulder muscles and return to the starting position.

NOTE: Keep your arms in line with your shoulders.

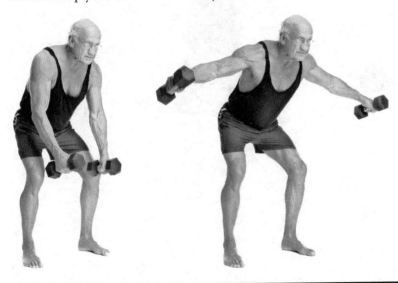

ADVANCED STANDING OVERHEAD BARBELL PRESS

Benefits: Works primarily the shoulders and triceps.

To start: Stand with feet slightly wider than shoulder width apart. Hold a barbell at the upper chest with an overhand grip. Draw your navel inward.

1. Lift the bar overhead until your arms are fully extended.

2. Make sure not to lock out the elbows.

3. In a controlled manner, lower bar back to the starting position.

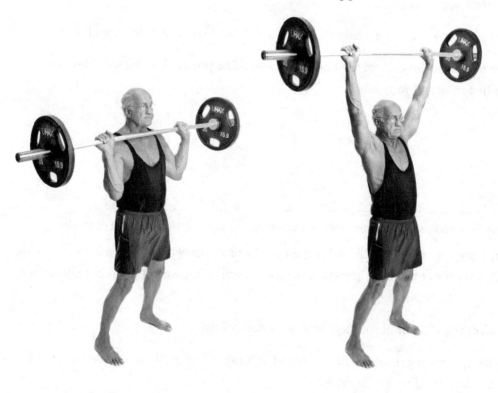

POWER PUSH PRESS

Benefits: Total-body exercise designed for power production.

To start: Begin with your feet a little wider than shoulder width apart, with a barbell resting against your front shoulder. Hand grips should place the forearm in a vertical position.

1. Slightly bend your knees and hips until the knees are at about a 120-degree angle.

2. Generate as much force as possible from your legs by extending ankles, hips, and knees. This exercise is an attempt to move the barbell in as little time as possible by using all the force you can generate.

3. The bar should travel vertically until arms are about 75 percent fully extended.

4. The rest of the distance traveled by the bar should be powered by the shoulders, which continue to travel vertically.

Legs

LEG PRESS

Benefits: This exercise shapes and strengthens the back of your thighs, front of the legs.

To start: Place your feet shoulder width apart on the platform of a leg press machine, turning them slightly outward. Unlock any safety devices and allow the weight to lower toward your chest.

1. Lower the weight until your legs form a 90-degree angle.

2. Drive up, pressing through your heels and keeping your feet flat on the platform until your knees are almost fully extended.

3. Try not to lock out any joints while performing this exercise. Return to the starting position.

BARBELL SQUATS

Benefits: This exercise shapes and strengthens the back of your thighs, front of the legs, and the glutes.

To start: Stand inside a squat rack, with a barbell placed on the back of your neck. Grab the bar with a grip around 8 inches wider than shoulder width apart. Make sure the squat rack is equipped with safety bars.

1. Lower your body until the upper part of your leg is parallel to the floor.

2. Keep chest up high throughout the motion.

3. Return to starting position by pressing upward, with the force mostly coming from the middle of your feet.

4. Stop just before you lock your knees.

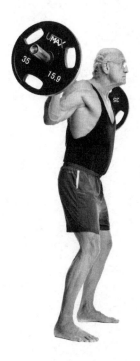
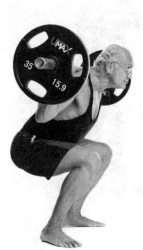

BARBELL LUNGES

Benefits: This exercise shapes and strengthens the front and back of your leg and tightens your glutes.

To start: Grab a barbell with your hands wider than shoulder width apart. Place the barbell behind your neck and draw navel inward.

1. Step forward with one leg. As your foot lands, bend both knees to lower your body. Your front knee should form a right angle directly above your ankle. Keep your torso erect.

2. Stand back up by pressing through your front foot. Bring both legs together.

3. Repeat through the first set, then switch to the other leg.

NOTE: Do not allow the back knee to touch the floor. As you lunge forward with your front legs, you should also feel tension in your quadriceps, and as you step back you should feel tension in your glutes.

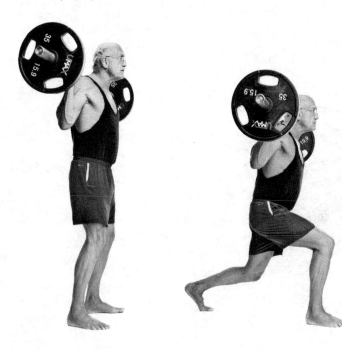

STRAIGHT LEG DEAD LIFT

Benefits: This exercise shapes and strengthens the back of your legs and lower back and tightens your glutes.

To start: Grab a pair of dumbbells with an overhand grip and stand with your knees slightly bent and aligned over your middle toes, dumbbells in front of your thighs.

1. Keeping your arms straight and knees in place, slowly bend at your waist and lower the weights as far as possible or until your chest is parallel to the floor without rounding your back.

2. Push through the middle of your feet and squeeze your glutes to pull yourself up.

3. Stop when your body is erect. Do not lean back excessively.

LEG EXTENSIONS

Benefits: This exercise shapes and strengthens the front of your thighs.

To start: Sit on the leg extension machine seat with your back firmly pressed against the pad. Draw your navel inward. Adjust the rollers so that they press against your shins. Keep your feet flexed. Grasp the handles alongside the seat.

1. Straighten your legs slowly to their full extension. Do not lock your knees.

2. Lower them to the starting position.

SINGLE LEG SQUATS

Benefits: This exercise will strengthen your quadriceps, hamstrings, and buttocks.

To start: Stand upright, arms at your sides, and draw your navel inward, balancing on one leg.

1. Bend at the knee until your leg reaches a 45-degree angle. Touch your toe with your opposite hand. Do not let your standing knee move.

2. Slowly return to the starting position.

DUMBBELL STEP-UPS

Benefits: This exercise will strengthen your quadriceps, hamstrings, and buttocks.

To start: Stand facing a step, bench, or box, holding a dumbbell in each hand.

1. Place your right foot up onto the step, creating a 90-degree angle with the knee.

2. Driving the weight of your body through your right heel, stand up onto the step.

3. Lower yourself, with control, back to the floor, left foot first, and step off completely.

4. Repeat on the other side (right leg leads up, left leg leads down; left leg leads up, right leg leads down).

LYING LEG CURLS

Benefits: This exercise strengthens and shapes the back of your thighs.

To start: Lie facedown on the bench. Place your knees beyond the edge of the bench. Adjust the rollers so that they rest on the back a little above your ankles. Hold on to the handles on the side, keeping your gaze straight ahead.

1. Slowly raise and flex your knees to raise your feet against the rollers. Your feet should almost touch your glutes.

2. Lower and return to the starting position.

NOTE: Make sure that you do not lift your hips off the bench, putting too much pressure on your lower back.

Benefits: This exercise shapes and strengthens the back of your thighs, front of the legs, and the glutes.

To start: Stand with your feet shoulder width apart and your hands behind your head, fingers interlocked and chest out.

1. Bend your knees and lower your body as if you were sitting back into a chair.

2. Stop when your thighs are parallel to the floor.

3. Return to the starting position.

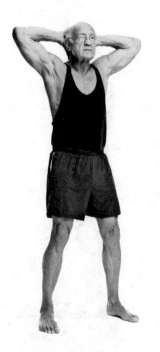
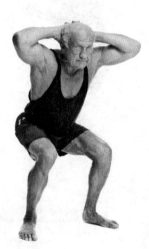

ADVANCED BOX JUMPS

Benefits: Develops power in the legs.

To start: Stand with feet shoulder width apart in front of a secured box or platform.

1. Bend knees about 45 degrees.

2. Jump on box with both feet.

3. Immediately jump down to your starting position.

4. Be sure to bend your knees when landing.

5. Repeat as fast as possible.

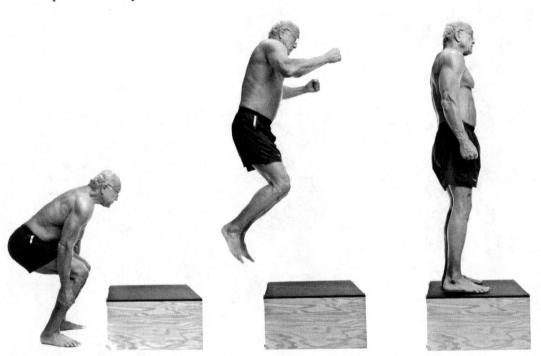

SQUAT JUMP KNEE TUCK

Benefits: Develops power in the legs.

To start: Stand with feet hip to shoulder width apart.

1. Bend knees to about 90 degrees.

2. Explode from bent-knee position into a jump. This means you need to generate as much force as possible from your legs by extending ankles, hips, and knees. This exercise is an attempt to move your body from a squatting position into the air in as little time as possible by using all the force you can generate.

3. Jump as high as possible.

4. As you begin the jump, raise your knees toward your chest.

5. Upon landing, repeat jump and knee raise as fast as possible.

GET YOUR SIX-PACK

The secret to great abs is not doing thousands of crunches every day. Focus your energy on getting rid of the subcutaneous fat (fat under your skin) that covers them up. To do this you need to burn the fat off your *entire* body. It is impossible to remove the fat just from your abdomen—there is no such thing as spot reducing (unless, of course, you want to go under hot lights and the cold, sharp steel of a scalpel). Fat is spread over the entire body, and I hate to tell you this, but the last place we lose it and the first place we put it on is, you guessed it, our bellies. So, train your abs like any other body part and burn the fat off your entire body with the right combination of aerobic and anaerobic exercise along with the Life Plan diets.

PREACHER CURL

Benefits: This exercise shapes and strengthens your biceps.

To start: Sit down at the preacher curl machine. Place the back of your upper arm against the incline support pad. Sit in an erect position. Draw your navel inward.

1. With your upper arm firmly against the pad, grab the handles on the bar, curling your arms up toward your face.

2. Squeeze your biceps at the top of the movement.

3. Slowly lower to the starting position.

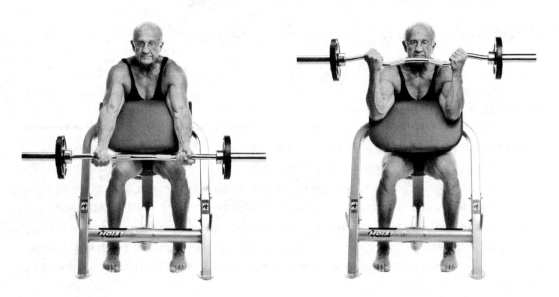

DUMBBELL CURL

Benefits: This exercise shapes and strengthens your biceps.

To start: Stand with your feet shoulder width apart. Hold two dumbbells at your side, with your palms facing forward.

1. Curl the weights up to your shoulders.

2. Lower them slowly to the starting position.

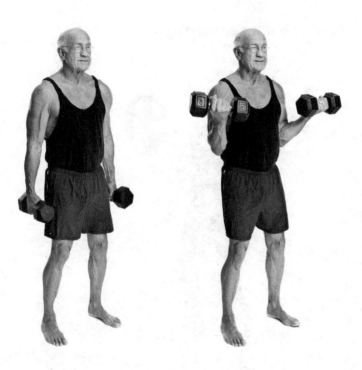

BARBELL CURL

Benefits: This exercise shapes and strengthens your biceps.

To start: Stand with your feet shoulder width apart. Pull your navel inward. Hold a barbell with both hands at about shoulder width with palms-up grip. Extend your arms in front of your thighs. Keep your elbows along the sides of your body.

1. Curl the barbell up toward your chest in a slow, controlled motion, contracting your biceps at the top.

2. Lower the bar slowly. Do not allow the bar to rest on your thighs.

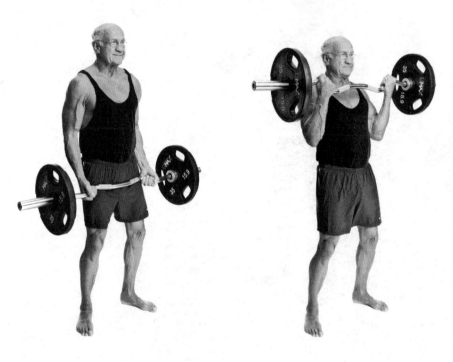

CONCENTRATION CURLS

Benefits: This exercise shapes and strengthens your arms.

To start: Sit at the edge of an exercise bench. Draw your navel inward. Keep your legs apart and feet flat on the floor. Grab a dumbbell and lean forward. Let your free arm hang to the side of your thighs, but do not lean on your leg.

1. Place the elbow of the working arm against the inside of your knee.

2. Raise the dumbbell straight up toward your shoulder. Do not rest at the top of the movement.

3. Contract your biceps and slowly lower to the starting position. Do not stop at the top of the movement. Keep constant tension on the muscle.

NOTE: For the at-home workout, perform this exercise while sitting on the physio ball or a chair.

CABLE CURL

Benefits: Exercise will work the biceps.

To start: Stand with your legs shoulder width apart. Grasp the bar attached to the cable pulley with your palms facing upward.

1. Keeping your elbows close to your body, curl the bar by bringing your hands closer to the biceps.

2. When the elbow is completely flexed, stop.

3. Squeeze your biceps at the top of the movement.

4. Slowly return to the starting position.

ADVANCED LUNGE TO CURL

Benefits: These exercises will strengthen your biceps and legs.

1. Stand with your feet hip width apart and hold a dumbbell in each hand with your arms at your sides, your palms facing forward.

2. Step forward with one leg and then lower yourself until that thigh is parallel to the floor. Simultaneously curl the weights up to your shoulders. Return to the starting position.

3. Repeat with your opposite leg.

Triceps

LYING OVERHEAD EXTENSION BARBELL

Benefits: This exercise strengthens and shapes the triceps.

To start: Lie on a flat bench with your feet flat on the floor. Have a spotter hand you an EZ bar and grasp it with a palms-up grasp. Extend your arms above your chest, then lower them to a 45-degree angle toward your head.

1. Raise the bar by straightening your arms fully. Stop before locking the elbows.

2. Lower the bar until you reach a 90-degree angle. Keep your elbows from going any wider than shoulder width apart.

3. Contract your triceps as you come back to the starting position.

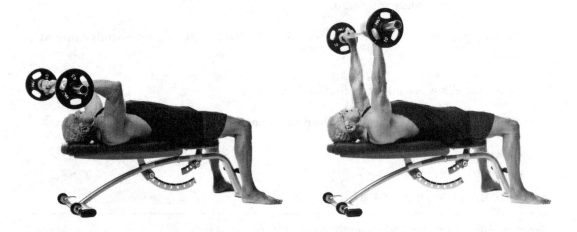

PUSHDOWN

Benefits: This exercise shapes and strengthens the triceps.

To start: Stand in front of a high cable machine with your feet shoulder width apart. Draw your navel inward. Hook a V bar attachment and grab it with a palms-down grip. Keep your elbows at your sides.

1. Press the V bar down with your hands.

2. As you pass the 90-degree elbow position, straighten your arms out and squeeze your triceps hard.

3. Slowly bring the bar back up toward your chest. Stop when your upper arm is parallel to the floor.

CHAIR DIPS

Benefits: This exercise shapes and strengthens the triceps.

To start: Sit at the edge of the bench, placing your hands by your hips, fingers at the edge of the bench, elbows pointed to the rear. Draw your navel inward. Hold your body up as you place your feet flat on the floor, knees at a 90-degree angle or legs straight as shown below.

1. Slowly lower your body toward the floor until you feel a stretch in your triceps. Keep your back close to the bench as you descend.

2. Push yourself back up and straighten your arm completely, contracting your triceps at the top of the movement.

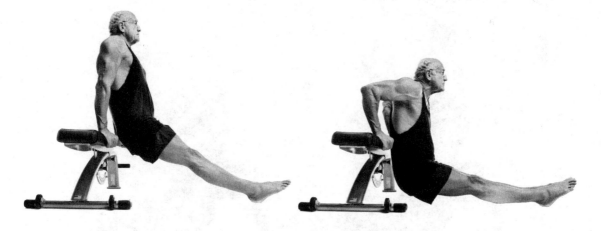

KICK BACKS

Benefits: This exercise shapes and strengthens the triceps.

To start: Stand with your feet shoulder width apart. Grab a pair of dumbbells. Bend at the waist, so your upper body is not quite parallel to the floor. Your knees should be slightly bent with your back straight.

1. Keeping your upper arms alongside your body, bend your elbows at a 90-degree angle.

2. Slowly extend your arms and contract your triceps at the top of the movement.

3. Return to the starting position.

DUMBBELL SEATED OVERHEAD EXTENSION

Benefits: This exercise shapes and strengthens your triceps.

To start: Sit on the edge of a chair with your feet flat on the floor, back straight, and with both hands, grab a dumbbell. Pull your navel inward.

1. Bend your elbow and raise your arms overhead. Keep your arms close to your ears and the dumbbells behind your head.

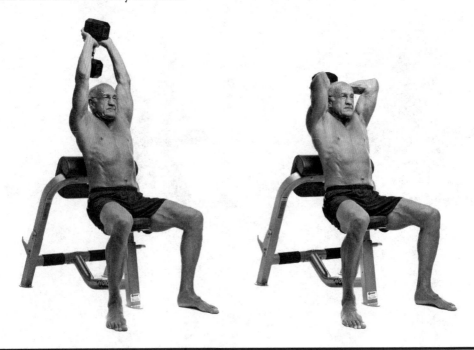

2. Keeping your upper arms stationary, lower the dumbbell behind your head, until your elbows form a 90-degree angle.

3. Press the dumbbell upward until your arms are fully extended and contract your triceps.

ADVANCED DIPS

Benefits: Exercise for chest, shoulders, and triceps using body weight.

To start: You need to find a dip machine, or parallel bars. Grasp the bar with a tight grip. Make sure you keep your chest up high. Bend your legs to 90 degrees and look forward.

1. Begin with elbows extended while holding your body in the air.

2. In a controlled manner lower your body by bending your elbows.

3. Lower your body until your upper arm is parallel to the floor.

4. Push your body upward to the starting position by using your triceps, shoulders, and chest.

5. Stop just before you lock your elbows.

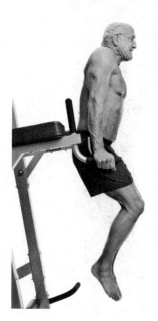
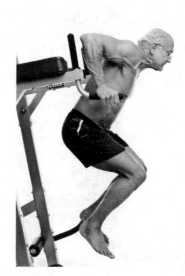

The following total-body exercises are used in conjunction with the High-Performance Workout. These exercises create a compound set system. An exercise that works a particular muscle group is immediately followed by a full-body exercise that has some emphasis on the same muscle group. For example: On day one a "barbell row, " which works the large muscles in the back, can be immediately followed up with a "crunch to jump pull-up," which will work the total body, with an emphasis on the larger muscles of the back.

WALKING LUNGE OVERHEAD PRESS

Benefits: This exercise works the legs, glutes, core, and shoulders.

Could follow: Overhead dumbbell press, dumbbell lateral raise, upright row, front raise, rear fly, barbell press (or any shoulder exercise).

To start: Grab two dumbbells and stand with your feet shoulder width apart and your torso upright. Be sure that you have enough space to walk forward about 20 to 30 feet.

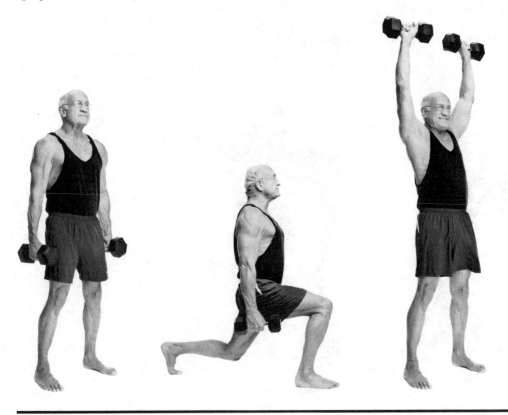

1. Step forward with your right leg moving around 2 to 3 feet from the foot being left stationary behind, and lower your upper body.

2. While keeping the torso upright and maintaining balance, do not allow your knee to go forward beyond your toes as you come down. Keep your front shin perpendicular to the floor.

3. Using mainly the ball of your foot, push up and go back to the starting position.

4. Lift the dumbbells overhead until your arms are fully extended.

5. Return dumbbells to their starting position.

6. Step out with left leg.

DUMBBELL SWINGS

Benefits: This is a total-body exercise and works all muscles.

Could follow: Overhead dumbbell press, dumbbell lateral raise, upright row, front raise, rear fly, barbell press (or any shoulder exercise).

To start: Stand with your feet shoulder width apart. Grab a dumbbell and hold it by the end plate with both hands. The dumbbell should be out in front of you and between your legs.

1. Keeping feet shoulder width apart, begin by bending your knees slightly.

2. Pushing your butt back and bending slightly, swing the dumbbell back, between your legs.

3. Use your hips and legs to swing the dumbbell up, over your head.

4. In a controlled manner, allow the dumbbell to swing back between your legs.

SQUAT CURL AND PRESS

Benefits: Total-body exercise that primarily strengthens shoulders, legs, and biceps.

Could follow: Overhead dumbbell press, dumbbell lateral raise, upright row, front raise, rear fly, barbell press (or any shoulder or biceps exercise).

To start: Grab two dumbbells and hold them at your side. Your feet should be about shoulder width apart and your torso upright.

1. Bend your knees until your upper leg is parallel to the floor.

2. Allow the dumbbells to hang by your side.

3. Using your legs to return to the starting position, simultaneously perform a biceps curl by flexing your biceps.

4. Once you are standing erect, lift the dumbbells overhead until your arms are fully extended.

5. In a controlled manner, lower the dumbbells to their original starting position.

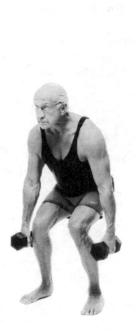
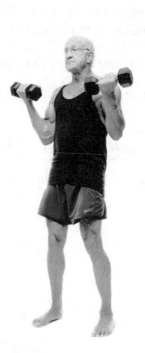
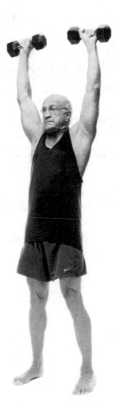

CHAPTER 7

The Life Plan Cardio Workouts

Aerobic exercise isn't categorized by what you do at the gym; it's differentiated by how much oxygen you use while you're moving. Oxygen consumption falls into three categories: aerobic, anaerobic, or a combination of both. Aerobic means "with oxygen" and refers to the use of oxygen in our body's metabolic or energy-generating processes. Aerobic exercise is any activity that increases the heart rate and uses oxygen while using large muscle groups. It also is maintained continuously and is rhythmic in nature for a prolonged period of time. Aerobic exercise is centered on endurance activities, such as distance running or cycling or distance swimming. Marathon running is almost a purely aerobic exercise.

Anaerobic means "without oxygen." This type of exercise consists of short-lasting, high-intensity activity, where your body's demand for oxygen exceeds the oxygen supply available. Anaerobic exercise relies on energy sources that are stored in the muscles and, unlike aerobic exercise, is not dependent on oxygen from breathing the air. Anaerobic exercise comprises strength-based activities, such as heavy weight lifting, all types of sprints (running, biking, and so on), jumping rope, hill climbing, interval training, isometrics, or any rapid bursts of hard exercise. Most exercises fall somewhere in between these extremes and include a combination of aerobic and anaerobic activities.

Kenneth Cooper, M.D., first popularized the term "aerobic exercise." Back in the 1960s, Cooper became curious about why some people who had excellent muscular strength did very poorly with endurance activities like long-distance running, swimming, and bicycling. He began measuring human performance in terms of a person's ability to use oxygen, which led to his groundbreaking book *Aerobics,* which included science-based exercise programs using running, walking, swimming, and bicycling. His book provided the scientific rationale for almost all of today's aerobics programs that are based on oxygen-consumption equivalency.

Aerobic exercise is also known as cardiovascular or "cardio" work, because it challenges the cardiovascular system and increases cardiovascular capacity by overloading the heart and lungs, forcing them to work harder than they do at rest. Your heart's ability to deliver blood (and therefore oxygen) to your working muscles and your muscles' ability to synthesize large amounts of ATP enable you to increase your cardiorespiratory fitness. The whole point of aerobics is to improve your ability to consume, transport, and use oxygen in all the thousands of biochemical reactions that go on continuously in your body—reactions that sustain health, prevent disease, and keep you from getting old.

When I slack off on my aerobics, I find that I lose control over my eating, even if I continue with my resistance training workout. I'm sure this is because without cardio workouts, my endorphin levels become low. Endorphins are opioid peptides we produce in our brains during exercise, excitement, pain, consumption of certain foods, and orgasm that produce analgesia and a feeling of well-being. Cardio also elevates my mood, enables me to handle stress better, increases my energy level throughout the day, and keeps me feeling young by helping me stay fit and lean.

Aerobic Exercise Protects the Heart

Research in heart disease and exercise published in 1999 marked a dynamic shift in our thinking about aerobic exercise. Before that research, the cardiology community believed that anyone with heart disease should rest, even prescribing prolonged rest. Now physicians are instructing men with heart disease to engage in supervised moderate-to-vigorous exercise. That's true for both prevention and treatment of heart disease. Aerobic exercise is important after a heart attack, angioplasty, bypass surgery, and heart implantation. The reasons are as varied as there are types of aerobic exercise.

We now know that regular aerobic exercise prevents age-related loss of endothelial function, the vitally important lining of your heart and blood vessels. What's more, studies show that exercise can restore damaged endothelium to healthy levels in previously sedentary middle-aged and older healthy men.

Consistent aerobic exercise also protects the myocardium (your heart muscle). Joseph W. Starnes, Ph.D., internationally known for his cardiovascular research, focuses on the association between exercise and its ability to help protect the heart during a heart attack as well as the effects of exercise, aging, and nutrition on the heart. Before his groundbreaking research, doctors believed that it took weeks or months of regular exercise to gain any degree of protection for the heart. Yet Starnes showed that even a single exercise session stimulates the heart to increase its synthesis of protective proteins, called stress proteins. Within twenty-four hours after exercising, Starnes says, these proteins increase enough to protect the heart against a variety of physical stresses.

However, exercise that is too low in intensity will not do the job. You must reach a certain threshold of intensity before cardiac protection is realized. Starnes claims that moderate exercise for 60 minutes can increase your protection greatly. In fact, he thinks exercise intensity above moderate improves the protection gain by only a modest amount. On the flip side, low-intensity exercise shows little, if any, cardiac protection. In short durations, exercise may provide indirect protection, helping to improve cholesterol levels and lowering blood pressure, but no increase in protective proteins is achieved.

Regular exercise training protects the heart from injury during a heart attack. However, Starnes's research also shows that exercise-induced cardiac protection is lost once regular exercise is stopped, which forces the synthesis of those protective proteins to come to a halt. In approximately a week, you will be back to whatever your pre-exercise level was.

Let's go over that again: No matter how long or how intensely you've been training . . . stop, and in less than seven days, you're almost back to where you started. You've lost your ability to make these protective stress proteins, and you've put your heart back at risk.

Aerobics Also Helps the Rest of Your Body

- **Burn body fat:** It is virtually impossible to reduce body fat without cardio exercise. While resistance training and correcting your hormone deficiencies will help get rid of some body fat, in order to really tap into your fat stores, you must do cardio, and do it for prolonged periods.

- **Increases resting metabolism:** Cardio exercise increases the amount of calories your body needs to carry out its normal functions throughout the day and night, long after you have completed the exercise. This is called your resting metabolic rate. The higher the metabolic rate, the more calories you burn every day.

- **Improves overall energy levels:** An increased resting metabolic rate increases your energy throughout the day, so that you are less fatigued during the day and have better sleep at night.

- **Improves sexual function:** Simply stated, the more fit you are, the better your performance is in bed.

- **Improves immune function:** Cardio exercise enhances key components of your immune system, which better enables you to fight off viral infections like colds and flu and even newly formed cancer cells.

- **Improves lung function:** Men may lose up to 20 percent of our vital lung capacity between ages 30 and 40, and by age 50, the loss is approximately 40 percent. Your lung function can foretell how long you will live, according to a significant Framingham Heart Study. Dr. Al Sears' groundbreaking work proved that if you don't challenge your lungs' maximum power, you'll lose lung power quicker, and prematurely age. Cardio training that involves short bursts of intense exertion followed by a rest period as well as longer endurance activities send a message to your lungs to expand. In time, your body adapts and increases its lung volume and power.

- **Improves nerve transmission:** Aerobic exercise improves the interactions of your nervous system with your muscular system, which results in greater strength, coordination, and speed.

- **Looking and feeling young:** A recent study published in the January 2010 issue of *Journal of Aging and Physical Activity* showed that consistent aerobic training had a positive effect on muscle mass, power, and strength, which could keep people active and independent for up to two decades longer than a sedentary lifestyle.

Types of Cardio

Aerobic exercise has almost an unlimited number of forms. Typically, it is performed at a moderate level of intensity over a relatively long period of time, such as by running a long distance at a moderate pace. If you include a few sprints in this run, you will be performing both aerobic and anaerobic exercise. Cardio exercises include running, swimming, racquetball, tennis, bicycling, rowing, resistance training with no or very short rest periods, calisthenics, martial arts, stair climbing, jumping rope, cross-country skiing, and fencing—the list goes on and on and includes any activity that increases heart rate and oxygen uptake for a prolonged time period.

METs Matter

Obviously, not all exercises are created equal. Each type of aerobic exercise uses a different amount of energy. In addition, all exercises can be performed at different intensities, and for different durations. In order to figure out what you need to do in order to maximize the time you spend exercising and get the most health and fitness benefit from the exercises you choose, you'll be using a standard list of metabolic equivalents, or METs.

A MET is a measure of how much oxygen we use in a minute when we are just sitting or lying down. It's another expression of VO_2. Or, stated another way, it's the base amount of oxygen we need each minute to just stay alive. It's essentially the same for everybody—3.5 ml O_2 per kg body weight per minute. A 2-MET activity requires twice the metabolic energy expenditure of sitting; three METs require three times as much energy as sitting, and so on. The maximum METs ($METs_{max}$) healthy people can achieve are in the range of 7.1 METs to 22.9 METs, depending on a variety of physiological parameters, including age, sex, genetics, overall health, and fitness level.

WHICH IS THE BEST WAY TO LOSE FAT—MORE EXERCISE OR FEWER CALORIES?

The only way to lose body fat is to achieve a caloric deficit by decreasing intake of food and by burning more calories through exercise. Aerobic exercise is a great way to achieve a caloric deficit. It does not trigger the starvation response, but it increases metabolic rate, increases all of the fat-burning enzymes and hormones, targets body fat rather than muscle tissue for energy sources, and increases the sensitivity of all cells to insulin so that carbohydrates are burned for energy and stored as glycogen rather than being stored as body fat.

Your maximum exercise capacity or $METs_{max}$ plays an enormous role in your overall health and well-being. A recent study determined that men on average lose 4 to 7 ml/kg/min (1 to 2 METs) in their maximum oxygen consumption every 10 years of their life—unless they do something about it! Men whose maximum exercise capacity is less than five METs are twice as likely to die as those with a maximum exercise capacity of more than eight METs. There is a nearly linear reduction in risk of dying with increasing levels of $METs_{max}$ (fitness). If you have heart disease and train to a point where you can achieve 10 METs, your prognosis is as good as that of those who undergo bypass surgery. If you can achieve 13 METs you have an excellent prognosis. Sixteen METs make you an aerobic master athlete; at 20 METs, you are an elite aerobic athlete.

In healthy men and those with cardiovascular disease, peak exercise capacity is a stronger predictor of death than risk factors such as hypertension, diabetes, obesity, heart arrhythmia, high cholesterol, and even smoking. Poor fitness is the deadliest risk factor of all! With each 1-MET increase in your exercise capacity, there is a 13 percent improvement in your chances of not dying this year. Men who can achieve exercise capacities of greater than 10 METs have a 70 percent lower risk of dying than those who achieve less than five METs.

Exercise capacities of 10 METs are the predicted levels for a healthy, fit man younger than 43 years old. The goal for each and every one of us should be to have an exercise capacity of at least 10 METs.

The table below gives examples of the energy cost in METs for various activities. This can give you a good idea of what you need to do to achieve the goal of having an exercise capacity of at least 10 METs.

METABOLIC EQUIVALENTS (METS) FOR VARIOUS ACTIVITIES

CONDITIONING EXERCISE

Bicycling <10 mph, leisure, to work, or for pleasure	4.0
Bicycling, 10–11.9 mph, leisure, slow, light effort	6.0
Bicycling, 12–13.9 mph, leisure, moderate effort	8.0
Bicycling, 14–15.9 mph, racing, or leisure, fast, vigorous effort	10.0
Calisthenics, heavy vigorous effort	8.0
Calisthenics, home exercise, light or moderate effort, general	3.5

Circuit training including some aerobic movement with minimal rest	8.0
Weight lifting, power lifting, or body building, vigorous effort	6.0
Health club exercise, general	5.5
Stair-treadmill ergometer	9.0
Rowing, stationary ergometer, general	7.0
Ski machine, general	7.0
Stretching	2.5

HOME REPAIR

Automobile body work	4
Automobile repair	3
Carpentry, general workshop	3
Carpentry, outside house, building a fence	6
Cleaning gutters	5
Excavating garage	5
Hanging storm windows	5

LAWN AND GARDEN

Carrying, loading, or stacking wood, loading/unloading or carrying lumber	5
Chopping wood, splitting logs	6
Clearing land, hauling branches, wheelbarrow chores	5
Mowing lawn, general	5.5
Planting seeds, shrubs	4.5
Shoveling snow, by hand	6
Trimming shrubs or trees, manual cutter	4.5
Gardening, general	4
Picking fruit off trees, picking fruits/vegetables, moderate effort	3

OCCUPATION

Building road (including hauling debris, driving heavy machinery)	6
Building road, directing traffic	2
Carpentry, general	3.5
Carrying heavy loads, such as bricks	8
Carrying moderate loads up stairs, moving boxes (16 to 40 pounds)	8
Construction, outside remodeling	5.5
Electrical work, plumbing	3.5
Farming, baling hay, cleaning barn, poultry work, vigorous effort	8
Farming, taking care of animals (grooming, brushing, shearing sheep, assisting with birthing, branding)	6
Firefighter, general	12
Firefighter, climbing ladder with full gear	11
Firefighter, hauling hoses on ground	8
Forestry, ax chopping, fast	17
Forestry, carrying logs	11
Masonry, concrete	7
Masseur, masseuse (standing)	4
Skin diving or SCUBA diving as a frogman	12
Police, making an arrest (standing)	4
Shoveling, digging ditches	8.5
Truck driving, loading and unloading truck	6.5
Typing, electric, manual or computer	1.5
Using heavy power tools such as pneumatic tools (jackhammers, drills, etc.)	6
Walking, pushing a wheelchair	4
Walking, 3.5 mph, briskly and carrying objects less than 25 pounds	4.5
Walking or walking downstairs or standing, carrying objects about 25 to 49 pounds	5

RUNNING

Jog/walk combination (jogging component of less than 10 minutes)	6
Jogging, general	7
Running, 5 mph (12 minutes/mile)	8
Running, 6 mph (10 minutes/mile)	10
Running, 7.5 mph (8 minutes/mile)	12.5
Running, 10 mph (6 minutes/mile)	16
Running, 10.9 mph (5.5 minutes/mile)	18
Running, stairs, up	15

SEXUAL ACTIVITY

Active, vigorous effort	3–4
General, moderate effort	2–3
Passive light effort, kissing, hugging	1

SPORTS

Badminton, social singles and doubles, general	4.5
Basketball	8
Billiards	2.5
Bowling	3
Boxing, punching bag	6
Boxing, sparring	9
Fencing	6
Football, touch, flag, general	8
Football or baseball, playing catch	2.5
Frisbee playing, general	3
Frisbee, ultimate	8
Golf, general	4.5
Judo, jujitsu, karate, kick boxing, Tae Kwon Do	10

Orienteering	9
Paddleball, casual, general	6
Racquetball, casual, general	7
Rock climbing, ascending rock	11
Rock climbing, rappelling	8
Rope jumping, fast	12
Rope jumping, moderate, general	10
Rope jumping, slow	8
Rugby	10
Shuffleboard, lawn bowling	3
Rollerblading (in-line skating)	12
Soccer, casual, general	7
Softball or baseball, fast or slow pitch, general	5
Squash	12
Table tennis, Ping Pong	4
Tai chi	4
Tennis, singles	7
Tennis, doubles	6
Trampoline	3.5
Volleyball	4
Volleyball, beach	8

WALKING

Backpacking	7
Downstairs	3
Hiking, cross-country	6
Bird-watching	2.5

Marching, rapidly, military	6.5
Pushing or pulling stroller with child or walking with child(ren)	2.5
Pushing a wheelchair, nonoccupational setting	4
Race walking	6.5
Rock or mountain climbing	8
Upstairs, using or climbing up ladder	8
Walking, 2.0 mph, level slow pace, firm surface	2.5
Walking for pleasure	3.5
Walking the dog	3
Swimming laps, freestyle, fast, vigorous effort	10
Swimming laps, freestyle, moderate or light effort	7
Water aerobics, water calisthenics	4

WINTER ACTIVITIES

Moving ice house (set up/drilling holes, etc.)	6
Skating, ice, 9 mph or less	5.5
Skating, ice, general	7
Skating, ice, rapidly, more than 9 mph	9
Skating, speed, competitive	15
Skiing, general	7
Snowshoeing	8

APPRECIATING VALUES OF METS$_{MAX}$

Super Athlete	National Athlete	IM Athlete	Fit Man	Average Man
23+ METs	18.6–22 METs	14.3–18.6 METs	10–14.3 METs	5.7–10 METs

Using Heart Rate to Estimate Potential Energy Expenditure

Heart rate (or pulse rate) provides the most valuable information about your level of fitness and your response to exercise. For each of us, heart rate and oxygen uptake are directly related throughout a broad range of aerobic exercises. If you know this relationship, you can use your heart rate to estimate your oxygen uptake while you are training. This is important information you will need to make sure you are training at a level of intensity that will allow you to achieve improved cardiopulmonary health, aerobic conditioning, and fat loss.

HR_{max} is the highest heart rate you can safely achieve. The most accurate way of determining your individual maximum heart rate and how it relates to your oxygen consumption is to have a cardiac stress test by a cardiologist or exercise physiologist.

Various formulas based on your age can be used to estimate your individual maximum heart rate, which will vary significantly between individuals. Your HR_{max} is biologically determined and declines as you age. The correlation to age is very strong. If a large number of 20- to 75-year-old fit individuals ran on a treadmill to exhaustion to reach their HR_{max}, the distribution of heart rates would range from approximately 200 bpm (beats per minute) for the 20-year-olds down to 145 bpm for the 75-year-olds. The most common formula used today is:

$$HR_{max} = 220 - \text{your age}$$

The generally accepted error in age-predicted formulas is plus or minus 10 to 15 beats per minute, and this is due to different inherited characteristics and levels of fitness. There might be some discrepancy when using the age-adjusted formula, especially for men who have been fit for many years, or older men in their 60s, 70s, 80s, or older.

Training Ranges: Heart Rate Zones and Rates of Perceived Exertion (RPE)

I believe that heart rate zone training is the best approach to all-around fitness. It works for a 72-year-old athlete like me, a 60-year-old with a family history of heart problems, a 45-year-old wanting to improve strength, or an 80-year-old who wants to be able to take the steps rather than an elevator to his third-floor apartment. It works for a 20-year-old who wants to drop body fat and become fit, a 30-year-old who has become sedentary from too much time in front of his computer, and a 50-year-old who is preparing for his second wedding (and honeymoon) and wants to be at his best.

The heart is a muscle that you can strengthen, just like any other muscle. And just like any other, it's a use-it-or-lose-it muscle: If you don't do cardiovascular exercise, your heart will lose its functional ability. Recent research has shown powerful benefits from exercising your heart in different zones, or rates of exercise, to get maximum benefit.

Heart rate zones are expressed as a percentage of your HR_{max} and reflect exercise intensity and the corresponding benefit to your heart. Once you have established your HR_{max} you can calculate your exercise HR for each zone that I have listed below. Your target heart rate (THR) is the desired range of heart rates you need to reach during aerobic training to enable your heart and lungs to get the most benefit from your workout. This range varies depending on your level of fitness and previous training.

Keep in mind that your aerobic capacity (endurance) improves much faster if you train closer to 85 percent rather than 60 percent of your HR_{max}, but some men don't have the capacity to start training at 85 percent, or they simply prefer to start training at lower values and gradually increase their intensity over time. Other men may even need to start at levels as low as 40 or 50 percent, depending on their age, level of fitness, overall health, and current body weight. The level that you start with isn't all that relevant. What really matters the most is that you get started and stick with it. Over time, as your endurance improves, you can gradually increase the intensity. Your body accommodates to both low- and high-intensity workouts by increasing the activity of respiratory enzymes and biochemical reactions in your muscles. Before you know it, you will be able to train at 80 percent or more of your target heart rate training zone and actually love it.

I think it is also important to compare your heart rate training zones with your own rating of perceived exertion (RPE). RPE is defined as how hard you perceive an exercise to be while you are doing it. This enables you to create a quantifiable method for guiding your workouts and determining your specific exercise intensity. Once you know what level of RPE you need to maximize your cardio workout, you won't have to keep checking your heart rate, and you can focus on the rhythm you have created or on the music, TV, DVD, or other interesting (attractive) people in the gym. It doesn't take long to correlate your heart rates with the RPE scale below. I used the example of the spectrum of standing still to race walking to explain the scale, but you can apply this to any type of aerobic exercise.

RATING OF PERCEIVED EXERTION (RPE) SCALE

0   Nothing at all, sitting or lying.

1   Very, very light: standing.

2   Moderate: walking down the street.

3   Moderate, no sweating: a brisk walk where you can talk at the same time.

4   Somewhat hard, moderate-sweat: a fast walk or slow jog.

5   Moderate hard, vigorous-sweat: very fast walking, jogging, or "power" walking.

6   Vigorous: running.

7   Vigorous-strenuous: a fast run.

8   Strenuous: a very fast run.

9   Strenuous-severe: maintaining a race pace.

10 Severe: race pace to win, last lap, balls-to-the-wall, can't wait to stop.

(Source: Modified from G. V. Borg (1982), Psychological basis of perceived exertion. *Medicine and Science in Sports and Exercise*, 14, 377–81. American College of Sports Medicine.)

The following list describes typical training heart rate zones and the rates of perceived exertion (RPE) most people associate with these heart rates. These will help you gauge the quality of your cardio exercise.

- **Warmup or healthy heart zone**—50 to 60 percent of your max heart rate (RPE 2 to 3). This is a good beginner training zone for someone who is out of shape or has existing heart problems.

- **Fitness zone**—60 to 70 percent. This zone will burn more total calories than the warmup zone (RPE 3 to 4). Of the calories that are burned, 85 percent will come from existing body fat.

- **Aerobic zone**—70 to 80 percent. This zone will strengthen your heart and is good for those who want to compete in an endurance sport (RPE 5 to 6). Although this zone burns more total calories, only 50 percent of them are derived from body fat and the rest come from glucose stored in your muscles.

- **Anaerobic zone**—80 to 90 percent. This zone will improve your $METs_{max}$ significantly (RPE 7 to 8). Drastic improvements can be seen in your overall cardio respiratory system, and you will increase your ability to fight fatigue. This zone burns only about 15 percent of its calories from fat during the exercise session, but fat calories continue to be burned for several hours after the session. Train at this level for 15 to 25 minutes to get maximum cardiovascular benefit. Getting to 85 percent of HR_{max} for 2 minutes won't cut it.

- **Max effort zone**—90 to 100 percent. This zone will burn the highest number of calories and is very intense (RPE 9 to 10). Most men can stay in this zone only for a few seconds to a minute or two at most. There is a high risk of injury when training at this zone.

Target Heart Rate Training Zone

The most accurate way to calculate your THR is the Karvonen Method, because it factors in your resting heart rate, which is another indicator of your level of fitness. To determine your resting heart rate (HR_{rest}), take your pulse when you are at rest—awake but lying down. The best way to do this is to check it three mornings in a row just after waking up. Add all of them together and divide by three to get your average HR_{rest}. The lower your resting heart rate is the more fit you are. Typical resting heart rates in men are in the 60 to 80 bpm range. Conditioned athletes have resting heart rates below 60 bpm. Lance Armstrong has a resting heart rate around 32 bpm. If you are fit, you should be below 50 bpm.

If your resting heart rate is greater than 75 beats per minute, you are 3.46 times more likely to have a heart attack, and your risk of dying is increased by 19 percent. If you have a low resting heart rate you decrease your risk of dying by 14 percent. These facts are all I need to think about to make sure I don't miss a cardio session.

Here is an example that will help you calculate your target heart rate training zone based on your resting heart rate.

$$THR = (HR_{max} - HR_{rest}) \times (\text{Training Range \%}) + HR_{rest}$$

Here's an example of a 50-year-old man with a HR_{max} of 170 (220 - 50 = 170) and a HR_{rest} of 60:

Training Heart Rate = 60% intensity: (170 - 60) x (0.60) + 60 = **126 bpm**
Training Heart Rate = 85% intensity: (170 - 60) x (0.85) + 60 = **153 bpm**

This individual needs to train at a heart rate somewhere between 126 bpm and 153 bpm to be in a training zone that will enable his heart and lungs to receive the most benefit. Ideally, you should wear a heart rate monitor during the cardio portion of your exercise, to ensure that you are at an efficient and safe heart rate zone.

Heart Rate Recovery

If you are fit and in good shape, your heart rate should recover quickly to pre-exercise level within two minutes after exercise. A healthy heart-rate recovery is a decrease in your pulse of 50 to 65 beats per minute at two minutes after you exercise. An abnormal heart-rate recovery is a failure to decrease your heart rate by more than 20 beats per minute two minutes after you exercise. If your recovery heart rate falls in the abnormal category, it could simply mean that you are out of shape and deconditioned, or it could be a sign of a more serious heart condition. While a general recovery heart-rate test can be done on your own or in a gym, you should have a formal stress test administered by a cardiologist if you are over 45, have a family history of heart disease, experience shortness of breath, chest pain, discomfort, or dizziness during exercise, or have an abnormal heart-rate recovery similar to that described above.

Your Cardio Goal—Burn 1,000 to 2,000 Calories per Week

The last piece to the cardio workout puzzle is: Just how much cardio exercise do we need? I have found that men need to burn 1,000 to 2,000 calories (kilocalories) per week doing cardio to lose weight and maintain great health. Just a clarification note here, calories are really kilocalories, but we Americans have simplified the term over the years to just calories. Whenever I mention kilocalories, you need to think calories.

You can easily calculate the amount of cardio exercise you need to achieve this goal. Let's use the same 50-year-old guy as the example. All you have to do is replace his exercise and his numbers with your exercise and numbers and you will have the answer that has taken scientists and exercise physiologists decades to come up with.

First, let's assume he is a runner and can run at the speed of 8.5 mph, which is 9.0 METs. Next, we need to know his weight, which is 180 pounds or 81.8 kilograms (180 lbs/2.2 lbs per kg

= 81.8 kg). To calculate kilocalories per minute we multiply the METs times 3.5 times his body weight in kilograms (kg) and divide by 200 (i.e., kcal/min = [METs x 3.5 x kg body weight] ÷ 200):

$$[9.0 \text{ METs x } 3.5 \text{ x } 81.8 \text{ kg}] \div 200 = 12.88 \text{ kcal/minute}$$

Our 50-year-old burns 12.88 kcal per minute when he runs on the treadmill at 8.5 mph. Now we need to know how much he must train to burn 2,000 calories (kilocalories) a week. Let's say he wants to do cardio 5 times a week, so he must burn 400 calories (2,000 ÷ 5 = 400) each time he gets on the treadmill. We know he burns 12.88 kcal per minute, so he must stay on the treadmill for 31 minutes (400 kcal ÷ 12.88 kcal per minute = 31 minutes).

There you have it. It's that simple to figure out just how much cardio you need to do each week to max out the health of your heart and lungs, and achieve a lean, fit, sexy body.

Types of Aerobic Training

Once you know which exercise you will choose, and the rate at which you can perform it safely and effectively, you need to choose the intensity at which you will train. The following are various types of exercise training that can be followed during your cardio workout. I believe the best of these is high-intensity interval training, which I have discussed last. You can choose the type that you like and will consistently perform. The absolute key to cardio training is to *just do it*, as Nike says. And keep doing it. If you get tired of a particular type of exercise, don't stop exercising entirely. Just change to another exercise or another form of training.

- **Continuous training:** Continuous training is cardio training that involves no rest intervals. It can be high intensity, moderate intensity, long slow distance, or fartlek training. Continuous training usually means working at 60 to 80 percent of maximum energy for at least 20 minutes, three to four times a week.

- **High-intensity continuous training:** This is continuous training at 85 to 95 percent of your maximum energy. This is a great way to develop your cardiovascular endurance. However, you need to mix this with some slower-paced training, such as LSD or fartlek (see definition below) at least once or twice a week to avoid overtraining and exercise burnout. You also need to have a good aerobic base and medical clearance before you start high-intensity continuous training.

- **Long slow distance training (LSD):** This form of aerobic endurance training is used in running and cycling, when you train at a talking pace. If you can't talk, you are going too fast. I do not believe this form of cardio is a good way to improve your cardiovascular conditioning and get rid of body fat.

- **Fartlek training:** Fartlek means "speed play" in Swedish. This is a form of conditioning in which the intensity or speed of the exercise varies. This type of training stresses both the aerobic and anaerobic energy systems. It consists of a 5- to 10-minute warmup, followed by a steady, hard speed for a mile or two, followed by fast walking for about 5 minutes, then sprint work until tired, followed by easy running, then full speed uphill for 100 yards, followed by fast walking for 1 minute, and so on. Fartlek training is a great way to get into tip-top shape and burn off lots of body fat. You must make sure your aerobic conditioning is great and you have passed your stress test with flying colors before you start this kind of training.

The Best of the Best: High-Intensity Interval Training

Interval training or high-intensity interval training (HIIT) is a form of training that is getting a lot of publicity lately. It is an exercise strategy that is very attractive to busy men because it improves performance with short training sessions lasting from 4 to 35 minutes. This is training that involves major muscle groups like your legs, back, and arms for people who are serious about dropping body fat and improving the functional capacity of their cardiovascular and pulmonary systems.

Dr. Izumi Tabata has proposed a four-minute form of HIIT that he claims is excellent for dropping body fat and increasing muscular endurance. I am concerned that cardio training of such short duration will not result in the production of cardio-protective stress proteins, which were discovered by Dr. Starnes and discussed earlier, and may not maximally improve heart and lung function and health. In addition, it doesn't begin to reach the 1,000 to 2,000 calories per week goal I discussed earlier. Until proven otherwise, I am promoting HIIT sessions lasting 20 to 25 minutes with a 5-minute warmup and a 5-minute cool-down period as the best way to achieve heart and lung protection and burn body fat. This is what I have been doing for the past year, and I can assure you it works.

HIIT is very physically demanding and isn't for everybody. If you have existing cardiovascular problems or other health concerns that limit your ability to exercise intensely, or if you are new to aerobic training, HIIT may not be right for you now, but you will be able to work up to it. It is not advised for the deconditioned until a stress test has been performed and adequate cardio efficiency has been developed.

This type of training is more effective for inducing fat loss than the longer-duration or steady-state cardio training methods described above. HIIT allows you to take advantage of excess postexercise oxygen consumption (EPOC), which occurs when your body continues to take in more oxygen after you finish exercising to replace the anaerobic work done (O_2 debt) during the high-intensity bouts of exercise you just performed. This is why after a sprint you breathe (or pant) until you have completely replaced the oxygen debt you created. By replenishing this debt of oxygen your body will slowly return to a resting state, keeping your metabolism high as it returns.

When you do HIIT exercise, you clearly get an extra bang for your buck, because EPOC also has a positive effect on resting metabolism. One experiment found EPOC increased resting metabolism by 13 percent three hours after exercise, and 4 percent after 16 hours. Another study demonstrated an increase in resting metabolism that lasted for 24 hours.

The definition of HIIT is high-intensity work alternated with rest or periods of low-intensity work. These bursts of high-intensity training are at the anaerobic zone (80 to 90 percent of max heart rate). During the periods of low intensity, your heart rate comes back down to around 50 percent of your max heart rate.

HIIT OFFERS ADVANTAGES STEADY-STATE TRAINING CAN'T PROVIDE

- Burns more calories while you are training and afterward because it increases the length of time it takes to recover from each exercise session (EPOC).

- Results in metabolic adaptations that enable you to burn more body fat.

- Trains both anaerobic and aerobic energy systems: The high-intensity intervals tap into your anaerobic metabolic systems, while the lower-intensity intervals use your aerobic system.

- Improves athletic performance.

I believe that another great approach to cardio for many men is a mixture of both moderate-intensity and HIIT. You can do two or three 35-minute HIIT sessions and two or three 50-minute moderate sessions a week. Mixing them up can make cardio training more interesting.

Interval training can be performed with any modality of cardio exercise and is very simple to do. For example, if you are on a treadmill or exercise bicycle, just start out at a low level, and once you are warmed up (3 to 5 minutes) advance the level of difficulty to 1 to 2 minutes of higher-intensity intervals interspersed with low-level rest periods of 1 minute. Just keep increasing your high-intensity level of work until you get to the percentage of your target heart rate you want to work at and stay there until you think it's time for a 5-minute cool-down. You will need a heart rate monitor to gauge the intensity of your workouts.

Most high-intensity interval workouts take around 20 to 35 minutes including warmup and cool-down. For each of the Life Plan cardio workouts, I've outlined exactly what this will look like. If you like to listen to music while you exercise, you can let the musical cues prompt you when to speed up or slow down. You can actually download onto your iPod fast songs separated by slower songs to create the perfect HIIT program for you. As your level of fitness improves, you can reprogram your iPod appropriately.

The Components of a Good Cardio Program

I perform 40 to 50 minutes of cardio four to five times a week on my exercise bike in order to stay lean and energized and keep my head on straight. However, I take one week off from cardio and resistance training every six months. This is the only time I miss workouts. This means no exercise at all for an entire week. When I return to the gym, I am really psyched and anxious, both mentally and physically, to get back at it. I'm not only energized, but I know that this rest period will help prevent burnout and possible injuries due to overtraining.

Just like the Life Plan for Healthy Eating, the cardio workout has three entry points:

- The Basic Health Cardio Workout

- The Fitness Cardio Workout

- The High-Performance Cardio Workout

Regardless of the level at which you are entering the program, the cardio component is built on the same principles. I use the acronym FITT to outline all of the areas you need to consider for your program.

F—**Frequency:** How many days will you need to do cardio work?

I—**Intensity:** If you want to drop body fat or improve your level of cardiovascular fitness, you need to train at a fairly high intensity. Remember to train at a heart rate that is appropriate for your goals. Start easy and increase your level of intensity gradually over several weeks to months. Remember, this is not a 12-week program, it is a lifetime program.

T—Time: How much time you spend during each cardio session.

T—Type: Choose two or three cardio activities that you like that can be switched around depending on your time and availability of training partners and facilities (courts, pools, gyms, and so on).

Your beginning cardio program may look something like this:

Frequency	Intensity	Time	Type
3 days a week	60–70% of your HR_{max}	30 minutes	cycling

After two weeks, revisit the FITT principle and increase your cardio program. A method that I commonly use is:

Week 3—Increase **Frequency**

Week 4—Increase **Intensity**

Week 5—Increase **Time**

Week 6—Change the **Type**

You can continue to go through this cycle endlessly to keep your heart, lungs, and circulation improving as you burn up more and more calories on a weekly basis. This approach will give you a lifetime of fitness and leanness you never dreamed possible. Use this method at each level of my Life Plan Cardio Program.

As your level of fitness improves you can move from the Basic Health Cardio Workout to the Fitness Cardio Workout and ultimately to the High-Performance Cardio Workout. Be sure to keep accurate records of your RPEs, HR_{max}, and heart-rate recovery. You will know when you are ready to move into the next phase of your training when your workouts become too easy, or your HR_{max} is lower, or your heart-rate recovery is faster. If you move ahead and find that you are not ready, don't get discouraged. Just go back to where you were, and in a week or so you will be able to comfortably move to the next level. Don't forget, this is not a 12-week program . . . this program is a Life Plan: You don't have to rush to the next level until you are completely ready.

BRET A. FITZGERALD

"As a guy, going from your 30s to your 40s is no picnic. But going from your 40s to your 50s can be downright traumatic. At least it was for me. I felt weaker than I had ever remembered feeling. I felt joint pain that was significant enough to use as an excuse not to work out. My shirts were tight in the middle and loose in the chest and shoulders.

Having been a triathlete from my 20s into my mid-40s, I felt like those days were over for me.

"The final insult was when I had to buy new pants, and squeezed myself into a 40 waist. When I put them on and they were tight, that was the ultimate moment of frustration, self-reflection, and truth. That was the moment that brought me to Jeff.

"I never thought that I needed to see a doctor about the way I looked, because I had been in the health club industry my entire career. I had a Masters of Education in Health Promotion from the University of Nevada, and had completed the Ironman Triathlon in Kona, Hawaii, in 1983 in 12 hours 39 minutes. But this time, I knew I needed help.

"From the first time I called the office to schedule my initial workup, his incredible team displayed total professionalism in a matter-of-fact, nonjudgmental forum. When we started together I told Dr. Life that I wanted to get back to my Ironman Triathlon shape. He was confident I could, and now I am really on my way. Since starting Dr. Life's program, I have gotten leaner, stronger, and more confident.

"For the last few years I was unable to run more than a mile. Now I'm running three miles. My shirts are now loose at the waist and tight in the chest, shoulders, and arms. I'm starting to train for triathlons again. Now I walk into a room full of 20- and 30-year-old guys and say to myself, 'I can hang with these guys.' This 52-year-old father of a busy 5-year-old daughter has found the modern-day fountain of youth, and he likes it."

The Basic Health Cardio Workout

Begin with 20 minutes, 3 times a week

Interval training basic

5 minutes warmup (light jog, low intensity, gradually increasing at the end of the warmup period)

1 minute moderate or high intensity followed by 1 minute low intensity (repeat 10 times)

5 minutes static stretching cool-down (see Chapter 5)

The Fitness Cardio Workout

Begin with 35 minutes, 4 times a week

Interval training intermediate

5 minutes warmup

30 seconds moderate intensity, 1 minute low intensity

45 seconds moderate intensity, 1 minute low intensity

60 seconds moderate intensity, 1 minute low intensity

60 seconds moderate intensity, 1 minute low intensity

90 seconds moderate intensity, 1 minute low intensity

90 seconds moderate intensity, 1 minute low intensity

90 seconds moderate intensity, 1 minute low intensity

90 seconds moderate intensity, 1 minute low intensity

60 seconds high intensity, 1 minute low intensity

60 seconds high intensity, 1 minute low intensity

45 seconds high intensity, 1 minute low intensity

30 seconds high intensity, 30 seconds low intensity

6 minutes static stretching cool-down (see Chapter 5)

The High-Performance Cardio Workout

Choose your favorite form of cardio and begin with 20 to 30 minutes of HIIT preceded by a 5-minute warmup and followed by a 5-minute stretch cool-down, every other day. The intervals can be:

- 1 minute moderate to high intensity followed by 1 to 2 minutes of low intensity, and continue to repeat this series until you are ready for a cool-down, or

- 30 seconds high intensity followed by 30 seconds low intensity is another option, or

- 20 seconds of high intensity followed by 10 seconds of low intensity

Here's what I do on my stationary bicycle:

- 3-minute warmup at Level 4

- 1 minute Level 9 followed by 1 minute Level 4

- 1 minute Level 10 followed by 1 minute Level 4

- 1 minute Level 11 followed by 1 minute Level 4

- 1 minute Level 12 followed by 1 minute Level 4

- 1 minute Level 13 followed by 1 minute Level 4

- 1 minute Level 14 followed by 1 minute Level 4

- 1 minute Level 15 followed by 1 minute Level 4

- 1 minute Level 16 followed by 1 minute Level 4

- 1 minute Level 16 followed by 1 minute Level 4

- 1 minute Level 16 followed by 1 minute Level 4

- 1 minute Level 16 followed by 1 minute Level 4

- 1 minute Level 16 followed by 1 minute Level 4

- 1 minute Level 17 followed by 1 minute Level 4

- 1 minute Level 17 followed by 5 minutes Level 4

- 5 minutes static stretching cool-down (see Chapter 5)

- Total time: 40 minutes. I do this 4 to 5 times a week.

The beauty of HIIT is that you can be very creative and design your own program that fits your time schedule and your choice of exercise. Changing it around also enhances cardiopulmonary fitness and fat loss, as long as you follow the 1,000 to 2,000 calories per week goal.

MAKE YOUR CARDIO WORKOUT FUN

If you're a walker, you may want to get a good iPod or some other means to listen to music or an audio book. If you're exercising inside, set up a TV so that you can watch it while exercising. Or you may just prefer peace and quiet. Do whatever makes exercise most enjoyable for you. You are much more likely to exercise consistently if you enjoy it.

The Life Plan Rigid Rules for Cardio Workouts

My "rigid rules" show how to make aerobic exercise sustainable, motivational, and transformational, whether at home, in the gym, at the office, or on the road. Since I won the Body-*for*-LIFE Challenge in 1998, the challenge for me has been staying on track. It is very easy to fall back into old eating habits and not exactly find time for exercise. What keeps me going is that I know that it won't take long for me to look exactly like my "before" pictures. In fact, I've found that many men who try to get a stronger, leaner body revert to their old habits and their old bodies within a very short period of time.

In order to keep going, I've developed reliable strategies I use to prevent my returning to the overweight, out-of-shape, unhealthy, unhappy person I was before the challenge.

- **Rule 1: Never miss a workout.** I count on a reliable training partner to help me keep this goal. There have been many mornings that I could easily have blown off the gym were it not for knowing that Rod, my training partner and trainer, was there waiting for me. I knew that the grief and abuse I would receive from him, myself, and others in the gym would be far worse than any pleasure I would get out of sleeping in! And I can also tell you that after I finish a workout, I have *never* been sorry I did it.

- **Rule 2: Promote a competitive atmosphere at the gym.** Now, I'm not telling you that you have to be a jerk to your friends or the other guys at the gym, but it makes it a lot more fun if you can get some buy-in from the men you work out with. I think this really energizes all of my workouts. Competition, for me, is truly a great motivator! I am always trying to set new goals and new challenges for myself, which really keep me on track. A little friendly competition keeps us all motivated. And when I'm working out at home, or when I'm on the road, my biggest competitor is myself. I have kept records of my performance over the years, and I am continually trying to beat my previous bests. When I travel and work out in new gyms by myself, I focus on beating my old records. This can be in poundage, reps, number of sets, or number of exercises. It doesn't matter, it's all about doing better.

- **Rule 3: Mix it up.** Cardio training should also be varied to make it challenging and cut through the boredom. For me, frequently changing my workout routine keeps my interest level peaked and my muscles always "guessing." It doesn't take long for your body to adapt to whatever stresses you subject it to, so if you want to keep getting stronger, fitter, and more muscular you need to change your routine every two to three months.

- **Rule 4: Always follow cardio with static stretching.** You must end a cardio workout with a cool-down, and the best way to do this is with static stretching exercises from Chapter 5.

- **Rule 5: Invest yourself in cardio culture.** I read all the medical, nutritional, exercise, and motivational literature I can find that reinforces what I have come to know and believe—regular exercise and proper nutrition enhance men's lives and improve their health and longevity. I don't have access to this information because I'm a doctor; I seek it out as an exercise junkie.

The Right Shoes Make All the Difference

Wear shoes that are appropriate for whatever cardio work you're doing. Most people, especially walkers and runners, wear their shoes far too long. Running in old or worn-out shoes is one of the most common causes of running injuries. Exercise shoes lose shock absorption, cushioning, and stability over time. Continuing to run in worn-out running shoes increases the stress and impact on your legs and joints, which leads to overuse injuries.

The easiest thing you can do to prevent those types of injuries is to replace your shoes when they're worn out. If you've been feeling muscle fatigue, shin splints, or some pain in your joints—especially your knees—you may be wearing shoes that no longer have adequate cushioning. A good rule of thumb is to replace your shoes every 300 to 400 miles, depending on your style, body weight, and the surface on which you exercise. If you weigh less than 175 pounds, you can get new shoes at the upper end of the recommendation. If you are heavier, you should consider replacement shoes closer to the 300-mile mark. If you exercise on rough roads, you'll need to replace your shoes sooner than if you primarily work on a machine, like a treadmill.

Mark your calendar when you buy a new pair of shoes or, better yet, write the date on the inside of the tongue. This will help you calculate the miles you have put on your shoes when you compare the purchase date with your exercise log in Chapter 8.

Putting It All Together for a Complete Life Plan Workout

N ow that you understand the components of the Life Plan Workout, let's put the pieces together to create one exercise routine that you can stick with for the long term. It's important not only to do the exercises and different types of workouts, but to do them in the right order. The following charts show exactly how this can be done.

The Life Plan combines all three modalities: flexibility and balance along with strength training and topped off with an intense cardio workout. Don't think that you've exercised by doing only one component: All three types are essential, because they work synergistically so that you can have better health, a better sex life, and a better-looking body right now.

I have tried many different schedules to complete this workout. I've tried doing it all at once and breaking out the cardio on either a different, alternating day, or later in the same day that I've done my resistance training. Any way you choose will work, as long as you get all three components in over a 48-hour period. However, for me and my lifestyle and busy schedule, I find that I'm best off getting the whole routine finished in one session. I exercise every day, first thing in the morning before I go to work.

The Life Plan Basic Health Workout Week

Mon-Wed-Fri complete

or

Mon-Wed-Fri without cardio, performing the cardio portion on Tues-Thurs-Sat

This workout program starts with a three-day-a-week commitment, unless you elect to perform the cardio on alternate days. I recommend everyone start at this basic level, especially if you are sedentary or if you have never participated in an interval training program. Follow the same exercise routine exactly for one week, making adjustments or changes on a weekly, not daily basis. Remember, it's important to end every session of exercise with 5 to 10 minutes of static stretching, so if you pull out the cardio section to do later that same day or on the next day, remember to end with stretching as well.

1. Cardio warmup for 5 min (bike, treadmill, etc.)

2. Flexibility—Self Myofascial Release (SMR) 5 min

3. Core/ab workout (choose 2 exercises from core/ab section) 5 min

4. Balance training (choose 1 exercise from balance section) 5 min

5. Resistance training—the Basic Health Resistance Workout

6. Cardio—the Basic Health Cardio Workout

7. Cardio cool-down: Slow down whatever you are doing for an additional 5 minutes

8. Postworkout flexibility—static stretching 15 min

Fitness Workout Week

- -

Mon-Tues-Thurs-Fri.

Resistance training in this phase is two days consecutively. For example:

Day 1 Mon

Day 2 Tues

Wed rest

Day 1 Thurs

Day 2 Fri

Sat rest

Follow the same exercise routine exactly for one week, making adjustments or changes on a weekly, not daily basis. Remember, it's important to end every session of exercise with 5 to 10 minutes of static stretching, so if you pull out the cardio section to do later that same day or on the next day, remember to end with stretching as well.

1. Cardio warmup for 5 min (bike, treadmill, etc.)

2. Flexibility—Self Myofascial Release (SMR)5 min

3. Core/ab—(choose 3 exercises from core/ab section) 5 min

4. Balance training (choose 2 exercises from balance section) 5 min

5. Resistance training—the Fitness Resistance Training Workout

6. Cardio—the Fitness Cardio Workout

7. Cardio cool-down: Slow down whatever you are doing for an additional 5 minutes

8. Postworkout flexibility—static stretching 15 min

- -

High-Performance Workout Week

Every other day.

Resistance training should be performed every other day during this phase to allow for appropriate recovery. For example:

Day 1 Mon

Day 2 Wed

Day 3 Fri

Repeat Day 1 Sun, and so on

You should be performing a total of 5 to 6 days a week of cardio during this phase of training. For example: If you elect to perform 4 days of HIIT, perform an additional 1 to 2 days of steady-state medium-intensity cardio for 30 to 40 minutes.

Follow the same exercise routine exactly for one week, making adjustments or changes on a weekly, not daily basis. Remember, it's important to end every session of exercise with 5 to 10 minutes of static stretching, so if you pull out the cardio section to do later that same day or on the next day, remember to end with stretching as well.

1. Cardio warmup for 5 min (bike, treadmill, etc.)

2. Flexibility—Self Myofascial Release (SMR) 5 min

3. Core/ab—(choose 3 exercises from core/ab section) 5 min

4. Balance training (choose 2 exercises from balance section) 5 min

5. Resistance training—the High-Performance Resistance Training Workout, including full-body calisthenics without a break in between

6. Cardio—the High-Performance Cardio Workout

7. Cardio cool-down: Slow down whatever you are doing for an additional 5 minutes

8. Postworkout flexibility—static stretching 15 min

Tracking Your Progress

There are many moving pieces to the Life Plan Workouts, so it's best to track your progress and record your personal program every day. Week by week, you'll be able to see how far you've come. The following chart can be photocopied or downloaded from my website: www.drlife .com. Fill it in after each exercise session.

Use the "notes" section to record how you feel after each component of the workout. This way you can capture the intensity of your workout, and your energy levels before and after. Some days you may feel like you are dragging, so it's a good idea to record why you think you are not at your best. You might find that your diet is affecting your energy levels, positively or negatively. Or you might find that you are taking the stresses of the day into the gym. If lack of sleep is a problem, you should record that as well.

You'll also want to keep track of weight lost and muscle gained. You can do this on the same form. Don't forget to take a shirtless photo of yourself every month. I promise you will be glad you did this when you hit 12 percent body fat.

At the beginning of each week, make sure to note the following:

- **Your weight:** Use the same scale week after week for the most accurate results.

- **Your measurements:** Measure the circumference of target areas in inches with a tape measure and record your changes in the grid: neck, chest, arms, waist, hips, thighs, calves.

- **Your percentage of body fat:** Use skin fold calipers to test body fat once a week. Calipers can be bought or borrowed at any local gym. Although they may be as much as 5 percent inaccurate, you can steadily see your progression, even if your initial calculation is incorrect.

DAILY WORKOUT CHART

Name of Life Plan Workout: _____

Day #: _____

Date: _____

Current Weight: _____

Weekly Measurements:

Neck: _____ Chest: _____ Arms: _____ Waist: _____ Hips: _____ Thighs: _____ Calves:_____

Weekly Skin fold test with calipers: _____

CARDIO/WARMUP: 5 minutes

FLEXIBILITY/SMR
_____

_____

CORE/AB	Sets	Reps
1		
2		
3		
4		

BALANCE TRAINING	Sets	Reps
1		
2		

RESISTANCE TRAINING	Sets	Set 1 / Set 2 / Set 3	Reps	Tempo	Rest
1		/ /			
2		/ /			
3		/ /			
4		/ /			

CARDIO	Distance	Frequency	Intensity	Time	Type	Heart Rate

POSTWORKOUT STATIC STRETCHING: 15 minutes

Establishing Goals

It's crucial to stick with this program for at least eight weeks. It generally takes that long just for your brain to create new habits, let alone for you to see changes to your physique. After eight weeks I am sure you will experience a level of enjoyment and pride from sticking with your program.

An important rule about exercise is its compounding effects. You won't get a lean, healthy, muscular physique in one workout. But you can obtain the body you've always imagined having when you are consistently working out and following a healthy nutrition plan. With that in mind, I find that the best way to achieve goals is to set reasonable expectations. Always set new, attainable goals every week.

First, define what you are trying to accomplish with your fitness program. Your goals can be losing fat, gaining muscle, sports performance, or even general health. A common system that is used for goal setting is the SMART system.

- **Specific:** Set a specific goal that you want to achieve that isn't too extreme. One goal could be to lose weight. First, set a goal that seems reasonable to achieve, like losing 10 pounds. Once you've accomplished that, move to a larger weight loss goal that is still within a reasonable range. A second goal could be to keep those 10 pounds off and lose another 5.

- **Measurable:** A measurable goal is one that you can objectively determine whether you have met. For example, make a measurable goal be to perform the Life Plan Basic Health Workout at least three times per week, with the goal of adding another day in two weeks before moving on to the Fitness Workout.

- **Achievable:** Make sure you are able to block out the time necessary to complete the Life Plan Workout. Work with your schedule instead of working against it, and make sure to schedule your workout into your daily routine, rather than waiting for free time to just appear.

- **Reasonable:** Remember, you won't look like me after just one week of exercise and dieting, no matter how hard you try. Modify your expectations to look for results after the first two weeks, and not before.

- **Timed:** Set a date in the not-too-distant future when you would like to achieve your largest goal. It may take you a few months to get there, but that's okay. Set the date in stone and don't change it once you have it set.

The Life Plan Food Journal

You should be keeping a detailed food journal in conjunction with your workout log. There is a direct correlation between food and energy levels, so comparing your energy levels with your nutritional intake on a daily basis is a good idea.

You should be recording the time of each of your six meals, the amount of food eaten as well as the calories. A detailed food journal will also include your level of hunger 20 minutes after eating each of the meals. This is a good way of tracking your satiety, which can assist you in learning how to eat based upon hunger and timing rather than habit.

The following is a sample weekly food journal entry. You can photocopy this form or download it from my website, www.drlife.com. Print these out and keep them in a binder to monitor your progress as you move through the different levels of the Life Plan for Healthy Eating.

Evaluating Your Progress

After you have kept your workout and nutrition logs for a few weeks you can begin to analyze the information that you have gathered. Your journals will offer you quality information on your performance and insight into why you are achieving your goals. So be very objective when reading your logs and ask yourself the following questions:

1. Am I progressing?

2. Am I working all muscle groups and at the right intensity?

3. Am I resting too long between sets?

4. Can I push myself harder?

5. Am I recording all pertinent information?

6. Are my energy levels good?

7. Is my flexibility better?

8. Am I eating the right amount of balanced meals?

9. Am I on track to reach my goals?

10. How can I improve in all areas?

DAILY FOOD DIARY

NAME: _____ DATE: _____ DAY: _____

GUIDELINES: Daily Calories Goal: _____ Approx Calories Per Meal: _____

MEAL #1 Food Eaten	Calories	Protein Grams	Carb Grams	Fat Grams

Time: Hunger level: Energy level: Totals:

MEAL #2 Food Eaten	Calories	Protein Grams	Carb Grams	Fat Grams

Time: Hunger level: Energy level: Totals:

MEAL #3 Food Eaten	Calories	Protein Grams	Carb Grams	Fat Grams

Time: Hunger level: Energy level: Totals:

MEAL #4 Food Eaten	Calories	Protein Grams	Carb Grams	Fat Grams

Time: Hunger level: Energy level: Totals:

MEAL #5 Food Eaten	Calories	Protein Grams	Carb Grams	Fat Grams

Time: Hunger level: Energy level: Totals:

MEAL #6 Food Eaten	Calories	Protein Grams	Carb Grams	Fat Grams

Time: Hunger level: Energy level: Totals:

Daily Water Total in ounces				
Daily Food Value Totals	Cal	Gm	Gm	Gm
Multiply by calories per GM		x4	x4	x9
Calories consumed by macronutrients		Cal	Cal	Cal
Above numbers divided by today's total calories				
Percentage of total calories		%	%	%

CHAPTER 9

Silencing Your Inner Demons

I have accomplished my health goals almost in spite of many self-created obstacles that sometimes derail me. If I get off track and eat the wrong foods, I eat way too much and face a major ordeal to get back on track. The same applies to alcohol. If I drink, I drink way too much. I have learned to recognize my demons: carbohydrates, fats, and vodka. Yours may look different, but whatever your demons are, we have to face them, eliminate them, and then move on.

Before I started my journey, my demons showed up pretty consistently, almost every day. But many of the men who come to see me have told me that their demons appeared during a time of crisis. For example, they would tell me that their life and their health were just fine until something "unexpected" happened, like a job loss, job change, residence change, remarriage, or divorce. Whatever the circumstances, change seemed to throw them for a loop. A year or more would go by before they realized how far off the health track they'd gone. Many gained weight, mostly around their bellies, their cholesterol and blood pressure levels worsened, sexual function declined, and depression set in. None of these triggers were enough to get them to see a doctor, until they realized that they were too tired to function all the time, or that their relationships were suffering.

What your demon is and when it appears really doesn't matter. My wife, Annie, a certified clinical hypnotherapist trained in mind-body techniques, has taught me how to get past whatever was causing my demons to show up. I learned that excessive food and alcohol were just obstacles I put in front of myself in order to hold me back from whatever I was really afraid of: commitment, confrontation, and sometimes even success. She taught me how to undo the damage I created within my subconscious so that I could make the changes necessary to my lifestyle in order to become the man I am today. More important, her work has allowed me to recognize the truth I had created for myself based on my own perceptions.

This chapter will help you learn how to lose the old programmed messages running through your brain, and help you find out what you really want out of life by using simple meditation techniques. And you'll learn how to get out of your own way with daily exercises that will help reprogram your thinking.

A Quick History of Hypnotherapy

Acceptance of hypnosis among the medical community grew rapidly in the 1900s with the practices of Dr. Milton Erickson and Emile Coué. Erikson concluded that each stage of our emotional development builds on the preceding stages, and each stage paves the way for the next stage. He believed that outside factors such as family, society, crisis, and environment influence the outcome of each stage of development. More important, the outcome of each stage is not permanent, but can be changed by later experiences and therapies.

At the same time in France, Emile Coué, a psychologist and pharmacist, introduced a method of psychotherapy, healing, and self-improvement based on autosuggestion or self-hypnosis. In working with patients, he noticed that remedies given with positive suggestion and repetition worked better than the remedies alone. He firmly believed that each person had the solution to his or her own problem: *"You have in yourself the instrument of your cure."* In other words, you have the power within to heal yourself.

Hypnosis was first approved for use by the American Medical Association in 1958. Over the years there have been significant advances in neuroscience to support and encourage the beneficial use of hypnotherapy. Yet for many years the media has portrayed hypnosis as an evil spell cast upon you by menacing figures whose sole purpose is to take over your mind and control you. These portrayals degrade the true value of hypnosis, spread misinformation, and create unnecessary fear and skepticism.

Hypnosis is a state of relaxation, and the hypnotist has no power over you. The hypnotist is simply skilled in script and techniques to guide you into a state of hypnosis. You still remain in control at all times. We know this to be true because we all experience hypnosis on a regular basis. We are bombarded by different forms of hypnosis every day without being consciously aware of it through the biggest hypnotist of all: the media. The most successful marketing firms develop advertising that appeals to your subconscious. This increases the likelihood that you will remember what they are selling or advertising, which in turn boosts sales.

Entering a Hypnotic State

Hypnosis is a natural, yet altered, state of mind. It can be achieved when one is relaxed and selective thinking is maintained. In other words, it is a state of mind in which intense internal focus eliminates external distractions, expanding your internal world and opening the door to your subconscious. Have you ever been driving along thinking about all that you needed to do for the upcoming week and suddenly, you arrive at your destination? You realize that you don't even remember most of the trip! Do you recall what you saw? How many traffic signs did you read along the way? How many times did you touch the brake or look in the rearview mirror? You were experiencing a natural form of hypnosis, deep into your thoughts. You were consciously thinking about other things while your ability to drive was unconscious. Your subconscious was fully aware of what you needed to do to drive safely to your destination. You did not have to consciously think about driving at all.

The key to a successful hypnotic session is your willingness to allow it to happen. Have you ever seen a stage hypnosis show where the subjects are dancing around performing crazy antics at the suggestion of the hypnotist? Frightening, huh? The truth is, the more willing the subjects are to allow it to happen, the deeper the trance, and the better the show will be—and yet, at any time, any one of them could "come back" and walk off the stage. A hypnotist cannot make anyone do or say anything that person is not willing to do or say. The hypnotist's job is to guide you into a hypnotic state or trance state and make suggestions. Each individual's subconscious is then able to accept it, or not.

The subconscious mind cannot differentiate between fact and fantasy: It is directed by visual imagery. The stronger the suggestion, the more vivid the image the subconscious creates. For example, if a hypnotist tells his subject to imagine that he is a ballet dancer, the hypnotized subject immediately "sees" himself as a dancer and literally begins to *feel* like one. In his mind, he has created a picture and an emotional response, and the subconscious begins to adopt it.

In stage hypnosis, the hypnotist makes suggestions that make for good theater, and the effects are temporary. However, in a therapeutic hypnotherapy session or during self-hypnosis, the suggestions are positive, reinforcing, and beneficial. The goal is to create a trance state in which the subconscious is fully open to positive suggestion. By creating achievable goals that the subconscious can read as visual images, the subconscious accepts these goals as already achieved, and then believes them to be true. That's where true growth comes from, and the ability for you to teach yourself how to achieve your goals.

We all have the power within to improve, to change, and to succeed. All we need is the desire to make it happen. The benefits of hypnosis are endless. This is just a sampling of the benefits I have seen my patients (including myself) attain:

- Become more focused

- Become more organized

- Control pain

- Decrease/manage stress

- Eliminate bad habits such as smoking/drinking/overeating

- Eliminate procrastination

- Get rid of negativity in your life

- Improve memory and recall

- Improve performance at work/at the gym/in sports

- Improve self-esteem

- Improve sleep

- Improve personal relationships

- Improve quality of life

- Improve sex life

- Lose weight

- Overcome grief

- Overcome stage fright/fear of public speaking

- Slow the aging process

Starting Your Hypnotherapy Program

We are all driven internally by *our own perception* of who we are. That is, we hold on to the beliefs that we have created for ourselves, about ourselves, from a very early age, which may or may not be the truth. Whatever that image or belief is, subconsciously it becomes our best friend, and drives us to happiness and success, or our biggest critic, and subconsciously sabotages everything we try to accomplish. The most common root cause of failure on any level in a person's life is poor self-esteem. This could have been caused by an event or events in the past that we may or may not remember or even be aware of. The event succeeded in implanting a negative self-image attached to a negative emotion in our subconscious, creating self-doubt.

The critic within each of us tends to have the voice of an authoritative figure such as a parent, a teacher, or a celebrity; someone who had a substantial impact on our development. It manifests itself as someone of great value to you during your development, who may have said something or done something that negatively affected you. Here's an example: You've done everything you can to please a favorite teacher. You turn in a project that you have worked extra hard on, expecting accolades and praise. You are already visualizing the cheers from your classmates. As you anxiously await her response, all she says is, "Class, look at the fine project that Bobby (not you) turned in! Isn't it wonderful?" Think of how let down you feel—she didn't even recognize all the work you did. There is no applause, nor the cheers from your classmates that you had anticipated. All there is is disappointment and negative emotion flowing around in you and all you can think of is how you FAILED . . . and how Bobby beat you.

Now, here's the important part—whatever the event, it may have been totally harmless with no ill intentions at all, but it was *your own perception* of the situation and your own hurting that created a false belief about yourself. The stronger the emotion, the bigger the impact, the deeper the wound. From that point on, every time that same emotion arises, no matter what causes it, you subconsciously put yourself right back to competing with Bobby and remembering feeling like a failure. The more energy and attention that is subconsciously given to the critic, the more powerful the critic becomes.

However, you don't have to stay in this rut. If you are ready to make some real changes to the way that you think and feel about yourself, then let's start by getting out of your own way.

Get Out of Your Own Way

So many times I hear the same stories: "I exercise, I eat right, I do everything I'm supposed to do, and I still can't lose the weight!" "I'll never look like him no matter how hard I try!" or, "It runs in my family—I'll just have to get used to the fact that I'll be this way for the rest of my life." *Well, it's time to get over yourself!* Negative self-thinking always leads to failure. You are in control and you already have the means necessary to achieve your goals right in your hands. But for you to effect change, making a change must have value to you. The first step to getting out of your own way is to make a list of all the good that will come when you start the Life Plan program. Stop wishing for it and commit to making it happen. Get a clear image in your mind of what you would like your body to look like when you reach your goals. The more willing you are and the more committed you are to your goals, the quicker and more effective the change will be.

Greg Got His Game On with Hypnosis

Greg was a high school student whose main goal was to be a better basketball player. He loved the game and practiced with passion, but he just could not make baskets. Instead of being on the court, Greg spent a lot of time on the bench watching his teammates play. He became extremely discouraged and began losing interest in the game. He had met Annie earlier in the year and knew that she was a hypnotherapist, and he asked if she could help him. With his parents' permission and his mother's presence during the session, Annie got to work. I was thrilled to see Annie's work firsthand as well.

Annie asked Greg exactly what it was that he wanted to accomplish. Greg thought it was clear and simple—he wanted to be able to score more points for the team. Yet through a series of questions Annie was able to reveal his real inner goal: If he could play better, and score more points, the kids on the team would like him better and he would feel more accepted. This was a huge discovery, because Greg was already extremely popular. But for him, being accepted by the team was the real value in his desire to make a change.

In the next session, Annie had found a video clip of his favorite basketball star in action. She had Greg watch the video several times and take notice of the movements of the player. Greg already thought he knew everything about this player, but Annie had him concentrate on the sound of the crowd cheering each time the player scored. Then, with Greg's permission, she guided him into a hypnotic state and instructed him to recall the video, which he did without a problem. Even though I've seen Annie work with patients before, the hypnotic state always amazes me. Typically, patients look as if they are in deep relaxation with their eyes closed, yet they are not really sleeping. Greg was no different—he was responding quite normally to Annie, as if he were awake.

She then instructed him to think about the video, and at the same time imagine that the player in the video was really Greg. She instructed him to feel the ball in his hands and feel the sweat running down his back as he dribbled down the court toward the basket. Then she instructed him to "listen" to the crowd cheering as Greg scored basket after basket. She reinforced that the cheering was all for him.

Even in his relaxed state, Greg's face began to change. He started smiling—at one point he yelled out "Woo!" and held his hand up for a "high five" as if he was celebrating. It was a phenomenal transformation to watch. While he was still in a trance, she asked Greg to describe how he felt. He was able to talk and stated that he felt happy, elated, and powerful! She then anchored this feeling in his subconscious by attaching a color to it—green. As she told him, she pressed firmly on his shoulder. She reminded Greg that green was his school color, and during a game, he would see green everywhere in the gym.

Annie asked Greg to remember that whenever he saw the color green he would recall the feeling of happiness and power, the same feeling he had at that moment. She also reinforced how loved and accepted he was and how he should accept that love because he deserved it. If at any time he started to feel unsure about himself, he could recall this feeling of greatness just by thinking of the color green. His final assignment was a bit of posthypnotic suggestion: Annie suggested that whenever Greg watched professional basketball games, he imagine that he was on the team and realize that he could accomplish anything. She then brought him back to a fully awake and aware state and made sure that he remembered everything that took place during the session.

Annie and I attended the next few games that Greg played in at our local high school, and the difference in his playing was really remarkable. He had more energy and passion than ever. He didn't make every basket, but he was scoring more than 50 percent of his attempts. Best of all, anyone in the room could tell that he was feeling good about himself, which actually was the real issue.

Hypnotherapy does not always work with just one session. The average is five to six sessions, depending on the issues that need to be addressed. Greg was desperate to create change, which made him a very willing subject. Typically, Annie will create self-hypnosis tapes or CDs for her clients so that afterward, they can use them at home for repetition and reinforcement.

Visualizations Can Affect Change

Visualization is probably the strongest component of hypnosis, and the easiest for you to do on yourself. Here's a little test for you: Quickly, don't think of a pink elephant! What did you see in your mind's eye when you read that? If you are in the majority of the population, you immediately saw a pink elephant in your mind.

Now here's one that involves your senses: Close your eyes and imagine a lemon. It's big and juicy. Imagine the color, the smell, and the texture. Now imagine you are taking a big bite out of the lemon—imagine the juice squirting into your mouth.

Most people will begin to salivate and many will pucker their mouths. If you did the same, you have just experienced what many call the *mind/body connection*. You can apply this strong connection to your own life. If you want a lean, muscular, and healthy physique, then start visualizing how you would look right now. Any time you think about yourself in this way, your subconscious will believe it, and you will be driven to achieve it.

Dr. Life's Best Visualization Tips

Here are a few more tips on how you can begin to use visualization. Before you begin, find a quiet place where you will not be interrupted and have a clear understanding of what it is you want to accomplish. Make yourself as comfortable as you can. Then close your eyes and imagine. Make the images vivid, be direct, and say your affirmations with conviction. You don't always need to talk out loud, but be specific.

Some examples of visualizations I have used are:

- I believe that there is no room in life for fear, negativity, or self-punishment. In order to get rid of them, visualize these emotions in your mind. Imagine them to be ugly little monsters. Confront them and kick them out of your life. Visualize them packing their bags and moving out, never to return. Then applaud yourself for a job well done.

- We often get worked up over little things. We need to learn how to let go of things that don't matter. You know what they are and what triggers your reaction. Instead, redirect this wasted time and misplaced emotional energy to areas that will bring value to your life. To do so, visualize yourself in complete balance. Tell yourself, *"My life is in perfect balance. I am happy and at ease.*" Visualize your family and friends happy and at ease because you are. Praise yourself for recognizing the good, calm person that you are.

- Teach yourself to walk away from dependent, addictive behavior. Visualize your healthy life without cigarettes or alcohol, or whatever your demons are. See yourself as a man who is always in control. Visualize yourself as strong and tall and walking away from all that you know is unhealthy for you. Recognize how good that feels. Congratulate yourself for how strong and in control you are and for choosing to be free of bad habits.

Using Hypnosis to Deal with Stress

Stress of any kind, if not managed properly, can have devastating effects on your health. Yet getting rid of or eliminating the stress in our lives through hypnosis is simply not possible. I cannot make your nagging boss disappear, or take away your mortgage payments. Managing stress through hypnosis, however, is possible. Annie has helped me change the way I deal with stress, and you can, too.

Believe me, I know that life is stressful. Stress arises from critical events such as the death of a family member or close friend, divorce, financial woes, loss of a job, a car accident, or health issues. The most common source of stress for men seems to be job related. I've also learned that some stresses begin as positive changes. Life events such as getting married to the most wonderful person, graduating from college, landing the job you strove for, getting a huge promotion with a substantial salary increase, and starting a family are all good things. However, each comes with a lot of responsibility attached, and with increased responsibility comes an increased level of stress.

The physiological effects of stress on our health are numerous. It can start as simple pain, a stiff neck, headache, upset stomach, backache, difficulty sleeping, and most dangerously, overeating. Soon, the body begins working overtime to combat the ill effects of stress, which then compromises our immune system and leads to chronic fatigue and sickness.

Simply avoiding stress or pretending it's not there is not the answer. Instead, I've found that hypnosis has been an incredibly valuable tool, along with proper nutrition and plenty of exercise. Here's a simple self-hypnosis, a mindful exercise that I use whenever I'm stressed. Do this exercise for 15 minutes at least twice a day. You can use this whether you are at home or at work. Though it takes only about 15 minutes, the results last much longer.

First, find a quiet area where you will not be disturbed. Turn off your phone. Soft music is okay but not required. Get in your most relaxed position—if you are sitting in a chair, place your feet flat on the floor and rest your hands on your thighs. If you are lying down, relax and rest your hands by your sides. Allow yourself to get as relaxed as possible. Close your eyes and take a few long, deep breaths. Inhale as deeply as possible, pause, and then exhale. Do this three times and with each breath, allow yourself to relax even more.

Now focus *only* on the rhythm of your own breathing and imagine breathing in relaxation, and exhaling tension. Imagine that each breath you bring into your lungs is a positive, calming energy that spreads throughout your entire body. Each time you exhale, imagine releasing any tension you may have inside your body—you know where it is—let it go.

As you become more relaxed, form a circle with your index finger and thumb on both hands (like an "OK" sign). This becomes your anchor, just like when Annie pressed on Greg's shoulders. Continue to focus only on inhaling relaxation and exhaling tension. As you hold your anchor, repeat to yourself (or out loud) several times: *"Today is a perfect day; I can easily feel calm and relaxed whenever I choose to; I choose to remain calm in all situations."*

Finally, acknowledge yourself several times: *"I inhale peace and relaxation and exhale tension,"* and as you say this, picture/imagine/or see yourself calm and stress free.

Afterward, whenever you find yourself in a stressful situation, make your "OK" sign with one or both hands. It will immediately remind you of the calm, in-control feeling that you experienced in your meditation, and you may find that whatever is stressing you out can be dealt with rationally and calmly.

Cognitive Restructuring Can Help Keep You from Overeating

In a 1962 article published in the *American Journal of Human Genetics*, James Neel coined the phrase "thrifty gene." He theorized that a gene, advantageous to the survival of our ancestors during times of famine and food scarcity, would be detrimental to our health today due to the prevalence and availability of food. Food is not only a means for survival, but part of our cultural norms. As children we were rewarded with sweets for good behavior or good performance. We quickly learned that eating food not only satisfied hunger, it made us feel good about ourselves. In some cases, food was used as punishment: "If you don't sit up and eat right, you can just leave the table!" or, "You've been so bad today you can go to bed without your dinner." Food then transformed from friend to enemy, which wasn't healthy, either.

Food is the focus of any family or friendly get-together, whatever the occasion. The first question we ask when invited to someone's home is often "What dish should I bring?" We have business meetings over dinner; we eat after funerals; the reception is the real focus of the wedding; we socialize over food; we buy food to watch a movie. I was on a major airline on my way home to Las Vegas recently, and the in-flight magazine devoted a two-page spread to teaching readers how to prepare themselves so that they could eat the most food at the casino buffets.

Often we eat food whether we're hungry or not. When we use food to comfort, reward, punish, or conquer, then food clearly controls us. Instead of nourishment, it becomes part of our internal dialogue. I call this "food talk." And, believe me, food talks to us all the time. But don't despair: We can replace our present destructive "food talk" with a much healthier "food talk" that is supportive and motivating and sends positive messages about our bodies, our well-being, and the control we have over our lives.

You can change your food talk by using a technique Annie has taught me called *cognitive restructuring*, developed by psychologists trained in the field of cognitive therapy. Cognitive restructuring is another type of self-hypnosis that has proven very successful in blocking dysfunctional thoughts. You can use a simplified form of this technique to change your own destructive food talk into a powerful constructive message that can become an integral part of both your unconscious and conscious mind. All you need is a notebook and a recordable CD player, a few blank CDs (or dig out your old tape player and blank tapes), and a microphone to record your voice.

To begin:

1. **Make a list of all your negative food talk.** Take a few days to do this. Talk it over with your significant other and your friends. Do the best you can to drag these thoughts and messages out of your subconscious. Remember, you already have the answers within yourself—dig deep.

2. **Make a list of all your trigger foods** (foods that you crave or typically binge on). Then write down any and all of the words and phrases that come to your mind when you think about these foods. Write down all the bad things these foods and uncontrolled eating have done to you. How have these foods and this behavior sabotaged your fitness goals, set you up for serious medical problems, promoted fatness and lethargy? Can you see that these foods are never worth the momentary pleasure they bring to you, because now they have made you feel so bad? They are literally killing you.

3. **Reconnect with the experience of feeling good about yourself.** Can you feel good about yourself when you don't eat these foods and can you control your appetite? Remember that emotion drives us. Breathe in that positive feeling. Write down how upset you are that your taste buds rule your life. The more personalized you make your list the better.

4. **Create a script** describing your particular problems and how you are going to deal with them. Keep it short, to the point, and most important, keep it positive. Avoid using words like "never, " "don't, " and "won't." Keep it present. Use phrases like "I eat only the foods that are nourishing and healthy" or "Each day I am leaner and healthier because I eat only healthy foods." Emphasize your goals and successes. Don't be critical of yourself. Always visualize yourself as the lean, healthy individual that you can become, eating only the right foods. Get creative. Add relaxing background music. Promote your personal strengths and include your short-term and long-term goals. Include all the key positive phrases you need to hear and want to etch in your brain forever. Repeat them several times. Reinforce your goals. Dispel all the mystery and attraction of the foods that lead you down the path to failure.

5. **Have someone you really care about read your script into a tape or CD**—especially if you don't like the sound of your own voice. Always end your scripts with praise and gratitude for the good person you are and how special you are and how successful you are. Listen to your CD several times every day and especially at night, while you sleep. Your subconscious is acutely aware and open to suggestion while you sleep. Be sure to listen to your CD before you encounter difficult situations like parties or visits to your favorite restaurant. It is through this process of repetition that you will ultimately and effortlessly replace your old food talk with the new food talk you have designed for yourself.

6. **Update or redo your CDs periodically** as you progress in your program or if they begin to bore you. Before you know it, and without thinking about it, you will have complete control over what and how much you eat, because you will have succeeded in reprogramming your brain.

Hypnosis and all forms of guided imagery are incredibly useful tools to help you achieve your goals. However, they are not a cure for clinical, physical, or mental health conditions. I have given you these options to help you achieve the best life possible. However, if you are currently under therapy for any reason, continue to seek the advice of licensed medical professionals as necessary.

You have now mastered two of the most important parts of the Life Plan: the healthy eating plan and the exercise plan, including exercises of the mind. In the next section, you'll learn how science and medicine have come together to increase longevity. You can change your health and support your transformation by following the right nutritional supplements regimen and by understanding the latest hormone therapy options. Both of these tools can help you achieve your goals to become sexier, stronger, and leaner for the rest of your life!

PART THREE

THE LIFE PLAN FOR OPTIMIZING YOUR HEALTH

CHAPTER 10

Why Hormones Matter

People ask me, all the time, "What's the downside to taking hormones?"

My response is: Your deficiency is the downside.

You may know that testosterone is the male sex hormone responsible for your favorite pastime, and I'm not referring to ballgames, pizza, or beer. You simply can't have sex without testosterone. But you might not know that it is also necessary for maintaining your high energy levels and vitality, increasing your muscle mass and overall strength (men simply can't build muscle without it), enhancing your ability to burn body fat (especially around the waist and inside the abdomen), improving your mood and emotional well-being, preventing bone loss, keeping your mind sharp, and protecting your heart. What's more, low testosterone level is an independent risk factor for both metabolic syndrome and Type II diabetes.

From age 30 onward, testosterone begins to drop 1 to 3 percent annually. Around age 40, it gets worse, and you will begin to notice. By your mid-40s, you start complaining about "feeling older." As a result, your work productivity declines, and you worry about the "younger" competition that surrounds you while your intimate life takes a nosedive. And as I experienced, your once-effective workout won't deliver the same results. Famed Harlem Globetrotter Meadowlark Lemon once described this situation quite aptly: "I run just as hard as I used to . . . it just takes me longer to get there."

Low blood testosterone levels can also occur in younger men—in fact it is now estimated that 20 million American men of all ages suffer from what is called low testosterone syndrome. This includes 2 to 3 percent of men in their 20s, 20 to 30 percent in their 30s and 40s, on up to well over 50 percent of men in their 60s and 70s.

Because the drop is slow and steady, symptoms of low testosterone are sometimes imperceptible until bigger health problems emerge. These are some of the signs that your levels are falling:

- Declining sexual and physical energy

- Decline in the frequency of early morning erections

- Decline in the number of spontaneous erections

- Disturbed sleep

- Emotional swings, irritability, anxiety, depression

- Foggy thinking, memory lapses

- Increased cardiovascular issues

- Loss of strength

- Poor skin tone and saggy, wrinkled skin

- Reduced lean muscle, higher body fat

- Weak bones, osteopenia, osteoporosis

This loss of testosterone and other related hormones in men is referred to as andropause, or male menopause. If you haven't heard of andropause, don't beat yourself up: Most physicians aren't comfortable with the term either. In fact, andropause is not universally recognized as a disease state. As a result, men are at a real disadvantage as they begin to struggle with symptoms similar to those menopausal women face: decreased libido, decreased bone density, fatigue, weight gain, loss of muscle mass and strength, and often depression.

When your LDL and triglyceride levels are high and HDL level is low, it's incumbent on your doctor to treat these conditions and get your levels back to healthy ranges so these abnormalities don't

ONE IMPORTANT INDICATOR

One of the telltale questions I ask patients is regarding early morning erections. If you can't recall the last time you had one or you don't have them very often, then read on carefully. Those early morning erections have nothing to do with the bladder, but everything to do with testosterone levels. With lowered testosterone, not only do early morning erections disappear, but so do erectile performance, libido, and sexual thoughts throughout the day. Ninety-five percent of the men who come to see me in their 40s through their upper 70s do not have erections when they wake up in the morning.

result in heart disease. In fact, if your doctor didn't respond to those lab values, he or she would be held accountable. And yet, when it comes to diminished hormone levels, conventional medicine doesn't accept the science. These doctors see declining hormone levels as a natural part of aging and strongly believe that you should "just live with" the symptoms and conditions associated with them. But if you don't have to "live with" heart disease or a broken wrist, why should you have to "live with" poor health, or a lower sex drive? The answer is simple: You don't.

Saying andropause doesn't exist is like saying cigarette smoking doesn't cause lung cancer. Just how many studies over how many decades will it take before our national institutes, medical societies, and academicians change their position? My position is clear: No man needs to confront aging and its related debilitating symptoms if it is possible to reverse them, or avoid them entirely.

Stress Shuts Down Testosterone

An important and often overlooked cause of decreased testosterone levels is emotional stress. Hundreds of thousands of years ago the "fight or flight" alarm reaction system possessed by our ancestors served as a major survival mechanism for very short-lived life-or-death situations. This system releases stress hormones with high catabolic activity, enabling our predecessors to rapidly break down body stores of fat and muscle for immediate energy that was essential for their survival.

We have all inherited this same genetic code, but today our stresses are rarely short-lived. Rather, most stress we encounter is prolonged and frequently perceived only in our minds: Few of us are fighting off a woolly mammoth. This chronic state of stress results in the continued release of stress hormones, which severely inhibits testosterone synthesis and may be the greatest cause of aging and the development of degenerative diseases such as heart disease and arthritis. That's why it is very important not only to keep testosterone levels within a healthy range, but also to do your best to minimize stress by learning stress management strategies and practicing the relaxation techniques that I discussed in Chapter 9.

The Body Fails without Testosterone

Testosterone is an anabolic, or tissue-building, hormone. A drop in this hormone is particularly serious because it is an early indicator of a disease state that should be addressed and treated. A man with low testosterone could face greater risk for heart disease, Alzheimer's, prostate cancer, frailty, and sarcopenia. The first signs of declines in testosterone are generally slightly vague: diminished subjective energy levels, increase in irritability, decline in mood, decline in cognitive performance, loss of early morning erections. While decreased libido and erectile quality are the findings most frequently associated with falling testosterone levels, they are actually some of the latest symptoms, with other findings present much sooner.

THE LIFE PLAN FOR THE BEST SEX EVER

Penile hardness tests show men having the best performance when they are:

- In excellent health
- Don't smoke or drink
- Eat clean
- Get plenty of rest
- Exercise frequently
- Maintain optimal hormone levels

Sounds like the Life Plan to me!

But even if you aren't experiencing any symptoms, a loss of testosterone is affecting your long-term health. Testosterone loss isn't just about declining sexual function. Men with low testosterone face real challenges with heart disease and early mortality, as well as other health problems.

Men with low testosterone have a 33 percent greater death risk over their next 18 years of life compared with men who have higher testosterone. ABC News aired a story in June 2007 about a significant 20-year study conducted at the University of California at San Diego, revealing how low testosterone levels continue to be associated with increased mortality.

The heart (myocardium) is the organ with the highest concentration of testosterone receptors. Testosterone is associated with several positive effects on cardiac health. It has been linked with reducing coronary artery disease (CAD) and hypertension risks as well as with improving cardiac function in patients with preexisting heart disease. In other population studies, low testosterone levels are associated with increased risk of atherosclerotic cardiac disease. Older men treated with testosterone can show decreases in total cholesterol and LDL. Low testosterone levels also are correlated with a greater degree of atherosclerotic obstruction when coronary artery disease is present.

The brain is second only to the heart in terms of abundance of testosterone receptors. Testosterone is associated with maintaining cognitive function, lowered dementia risk, and decreasing symptoms of depression, anxiety, and panic disorders. Maintained healthy testosterone levels carry a significant cognitive benefit.

Finally, diminished hormones, particularly testosterone, put men at risk for debilitating diseases caused by osteoporosis, such as hip fractures. In addition to declining bone density, low testosterone levels are linked with muscle loss. Studies have been done looking at the relationship between testosterone replacement and a return to a more favorable body composition. The consensus from the medical literature to date is that testosterone supplementation is accompanied by gains in lean mass across all age groups. It is associated with reduced body fat, with some preferential fat loss seen on the abdomen.

Testosterone, Erectile Function, and Libido

The effects of testosterone on erectile function and libido have been well documented. Therapies that restore natural testosterone levels show real improvement on several sexual performance fronts. In studies of sexual function, mood, and well-being, testosterone levels and supplementation correlate with improved quality of life. That should be no surprise: What man would not be in a better mood if he was having better sex?

An estimated 34 percent of all American men (ages 40 to 70) suffer from some significant level of erectile dysfunction (ED). Worse, one of the first signs of heart disease is diminished penile hardness. In fact, research has shown that men experience ED four or five years before a heart attack. ED is also an early warning of:

- High cholesterol (especially LDL-C, low-density lipoprotein cholesterol)

- Hypertension

- Depression/stress

- Obesity

Don't get trapped in the denial game. Talk to your doctor if you're having problems with sexual function, not only to regain your intimate life and self-esteem, but also to improve your overall health. I agree with the findings of a December 2010 study from Brown University, which recommends that all men, beginning at age 40, be screened annually for low serum testosterone levels.

Meet Charlie

Charlie is a 49-year-old ophthalmologist who was 60 pounds overweight with a 46½ inch waist, very high cholesterol levels, early osteoporosis, and the beginning of type 2 diabetes. He was deficient in testosterone, DHEA, and growth hormone. He complained about a loss of energy, no sex drive, a loss of interest in his medical practice, a deteriorating relationship with his wife, mild depression, and a loss of joy and purpose in his life.

I had Charlie start following the Life Plan diet and exercise program. His deficient hormones were augmented to healthy levels and monitored on a regular basis. At his three-month followup evaluation Charlie had already lost 28 pounds of body fat and gained 5 pounds of muscle. He told me that his energy levels had dramatically increased, and all aspects of his life had improved. One year later he was still following my program, and had dropped his body fat from 42.5 down to 18 percent.

The Truth About Testosterone and Prostate Cancer Risk

Most physicians I meet have got it all wrong when it comes to prostate cancer and testosterone. While testosterone is associated with prostate cancer risk, it is in the exact opposite relationship than they believe. Historically, doctors feared that raising testosterone levels might cause prostate cancer to grow. This fear stems from a 1941 journal article reporting that testosterone injections caused an enhanced rate of prostate growth and castration caused prostate regression. Unfortunately, this study was conducted on *one* patient. Further science, however, has failed to support this review. Another large longitudinal study found no relationship between testosterone concentrations and the risk for prostate cancer, except to find that one risk factor of prostate cancer was low testosterone, not high.

My Decision

Five years after winning the 1998 Body-*for*-LIFE contest, I found that I was gaining body fat and losing strength, despite eating clean and exercising vigorously. Then I was introduced to age management medicine via the Cenegenics Medical Institute and realized diminished hormones might be part of my problem. Diagnostics revealed my testosterone levels were below the reference range. So I took my own advice and my age management physician started me on testosterone therapy. I've never looked back.

Within two months I began feeling a remarkable change: more strength, gains in muscle mass, improved sexual function, higher energy levels, reduced cholesterol, good blood sugar control, clearer thinking, and a zest for life. I know that there's no way I could accomplish all that I do today at 72 without correcting my hormone deficiencies, eating healthy, and exercising right. But that's me. You have to examine your own health issues and goals. I'm here to help you in that journey, whatever direction you choose.

WHAT'S THE DIFFERENCE BETWEEN CORRECTING HORMONE DEFICIENCIES AND TESTOSTERONE ABUSE AMONG BODYBUILDERS AND ATHLETES?

Bodybuilders and athletes may use testosterone replacement therapy, but they use it illegally. They may not have a clinically proven hormone deficiency and are using the drug only for illegal performance enhancement. In fact, many athletes purposely don't get blood work drawn to avoid any medical record of their use. Without the right screening, these men have no idea what their pretreatment levels were. I suspect that many bodybuilders and athletes who illegally use testosterone have testosterone levels 10 to 20 times higher than the top end of the normal reference range. And because they don't get periodic blood work to monitor levels, they can suffer from testosterone's breakdown products or dangerous side effects.

Testosterone Therapies Are Safe and Effective

Supplementing sex hormones in men with low testosterone levels has been discouraged by most of the medical community because they believed it was unnatural and put men at risk for disease. In the last few years this thinking has started to change as a result of numerous recent scientific studies showing just the opposite.

In recent years, the pharmaceutical industry has come up with novel methods of administering natural testosterone. Side effects typically occur during the first few months, but usually resolve themselves. These can include skin reactions such as acne, oily skin, breast tenderness, erythrocytosis (increased production of red blood cells), COPD (chronic obstructive pulmonary disease), sleep apnea, and lower extremity edema (swelling). Talk to your doctor about the following treatment options if you think you are a candidate for this type of therapy:

- **Transdermal—gels, creams, or patches.** I'm not a fan of this approach. Its absorption can be affected by weather conditions, and it can be transferred to your partner, or even your kids or grandkids. Plus, you need to apply it daily.

- **Pellets—surgically implanted into your muscles.** This testosterone delivery method slowly leaks into your system as it dissolves over a period of weeks. Problems arise if levels become too high; you'll need to have a pellet taken out. Low levels mean another pellet needs to be inserted.

- **Human chorionic gonadotropin injection.** While this method works great for younger men with viable, healthy testicles, it's less effective for the 50-plus crowd. This therapy, which is injected at the abdomen, stimulates the testicles to create more testosterone on their own.

- **Weekly intramuscular injections.** This is my preferred method, because it provides a more steady state of testosterone in the bloodstream.

Increasing Testosterone Naturally

Before you rush out to your doctor's office, there are a few very important things you need to know. Testosterone replacement therapy is not for everyone—many of you can achieve the same results naturally by changing your lifestyle! There are many things we can all do to increase our levels of testosterone without the help of the pharmaceutical industry.

The first is improving your eating habits by following the Life Plan. Proper nutrition plays an all-important role in keeping testosterone levels up. Men must eat plenty of protein, because protein stimulates the hormone glucagon and the muscle-building responses important for testosterone release. Also eat more vegetables and nontropical fruit (skip the bananas and pineapple) and be sure to greatly limit the intake of simple sugars and starches (high-glycemic-index carbs). Since they create a state of chronically elevated levels of insulin and cortisol, these hormones oppose the action of testosterone and interfere with its production. Also, don't forget about essential fatty acids (omega-3s) found in fish and flaxseed as well as some saturated fats. These nutrients are essential for the body to produce testosterone. Studies clearly show that low-fat diets result in low testosterone levels, and diets higher in protein, lower in carbohydrates, and moderate in fats result in the greatest sustained high levels of testosterone. If your diet is low in fat and protein and high in complex carbohydrates and fiber, your testosterone level will remain very low, and you will never be able to build muscle mass and strength no matter how hard you train.

TESTOSTERONE DELIVERY METHODS

- Topical (daily)

- Under the tongue (twice daily)

- Intramuscularly (weekly or twice weekly)

- Subcutaneous T Implants (T pellets/depot T) once every 3 to 6 months

The next area of importance is exercise. Both the lack of physical activity and excessive physical activity (overtraining) will decrease your testosterone level. It is the duration, intensity, and frequency of exercise that determine testosterone levels. Testosterone levels increase the most when the exercise is short and very intense. It's the core exercises, such as squats and bench presses, that train large muscle groups and do the best job of raising testosterone. This explains why squats help build upper-body muscles.

Testosterone actually decreases during extended periods of endurance training. After 60 minutes of exercise, cortisol levels begin to rise and testosterone levels decrease as a result of overtraining. This decrease can last up to six days. For this reason, some men who follow my program split their training sessions up and don't perform aerobic training during the same session that they lift weights. If your testosterone levels are not an issue, then you don't have to split your training.

Finally, make sure you get a full eight hours of sleep as often as possible to maximize your testosterone production. Hormone production is greatest when your body is at rest, which is why it's important to get good sleep.

Kegels for Men

For the average man, foreplay takes between three to six minutes, while orgasms last on average 10 to 16 seconds. In order to up your average without upping your testosterone, exercise your pelvic floor muscles (PC) with Kegels. Aging, obesity/overweight, and weak connective tissue all put stress on your pelvic floor muscles and weaken them. The goal is to strengthen the PC to achieve better sexual gratification, by making your erections stronger and harder with more ejaculatory control.

Research by urologist Dr. Frank Sommer demonstrated that men doing PC exercises had 80 percent stronger, harder erections—performing better than those taking erectile dysfunction medications such as Viagra. Another study, led by Dr. Grace Dorey, showed that 40 percent of men who learned how to do Kegels were completely cured of ED and 35 percent had significant improvement.

Step one: Find your PC muscle. What you don't want to do is squeeze the wrong muscle. Here's a simple way to make sure you have it right: The next time you have to urinate, stop your flow midstream. The muscles you use to do that are part of the PC. But don't make this a habit, because interrupting urine flow can cause bladder problems.

Variations with 5 to 10 minute sessions. Start at 10 reps and increase to 20 to 30 reps, repeating several times a day. It will take three to four weeks to notice a difference.

Slow Kegels: Tighten the PC, holding for a slow count of 3; relax and repeat 10 times.

Quick Kegels: Tighten the PC and relax as many times as you can in 10 seconds.

Big move Kegels: Tighten your entire abdomen and PC, then force the pressure outward by bearing down.

Fluttering Kegels: Quickly tighten and relax the PC using a fluttering movement for 1 to 5 seconds, then repeat.

Other Hormones to Consider

- -

There is a wide range of bioidentical hormones that you can consider replacing, depending on your current health status and deficiencies you may have. However, not all hormone therapies are the same. Synthetic hormones like methyltestosterone carry a black box warning connecting it to liver cancer. It has also been shown that growth hormones from cadavers cause cancer. I prescribe only pharmaceutically approved hormones, which are plant-based, natural, and safe. These hormones produce the same physiological responses as the body's natural hormones.

Besides testosterone, the other hormones I most commonly prescribe for men are DHEA, thyroid hormone, melatonin, and on rare occasions, growth hormone after appropriate testing (see Chapter 11).

- **DHEA (Dehydroepiandrosterone)** is produced in the adrenal cortex of the brain as well as the testes. It is then converted to estrogen and testosterone. Reestablishing DHEA balance to more youthful levels can enhance sexual desire, performance, and overall mood. It is also used for increasing production of your own growth hormone, combating chronic fatigue syndrome, depression, memory loss, and osteoporosis, and protecting the body from the ravages of age. This can be purchased over the counter as a supplement, but I recommend pharmaceutical-grade DHEA to make sure you are really getting what you are paying for. I have tested many of my patients taking inferior DHEA products and found surprisingly low blood levels.

- **Thyroid (T3 and/or T4):** Some men experiencing sexual dysfunction may actually have underlying thyroid disease, and feel better on a combination of the hormones T4 and T3. Your thyroid produces T4 and then your body converts it to T3, a more active form. These hormones can also help relieve depression, brain fog, fatigue, and other age-related symptoms. They can be obtained with a doctor's prescription after determining a deficiency by a simple blood test.

- **Melatonin:** You may have heard that supplementing with melatonin helps regulate sleep patterns, but it also has antioxidant properties for overall health. Melatonin can help you relax, so it may also improve sexual performance. This can be purchased over the counter as a supplement.

Creating a Life Plan

I believe that most older men could benefit from this therapy, as could many younger men in their 40s and 50s, and even some in their 30s. You will need to work with your current physician to come up with a program that optimizes your hormone levels. A total serum testosterone test done first thing in the morning is necessary to determine your current levels. Some specialists believe that they also need to know the free or unbound testosterone level to get a true estimate of testosterone status. The normal range for total testosterone is between 300 and 1,000 nanograms per deciliter. Levels between 200 and 300 ng/dl are considered to be borderline, and levels below 200 ng/dl indicate a clear deficiency.

If your test comes back with a testosterone level in the 100 to 200 range, a traditional doctor may say, "Well, Joe, you're okay . . . you're in the normal range." What he or she isn't saying is that low-range normal is the equivalent of getting a D-minus on your report card. I don't want to be a low-grade anything. I want to be at the top of my game, especially when it comes to two very important parts of my life: my health and sex. Staying in the upper normal range means having a testosterone level of 900, 1,000, or even 1,100.

If you have borderline or even very low testosterone levels, you can first try to raise your levels through exercise, weight loss, proper nutrition, supplementation, avoiding smoking, minimizing the use of alcohol, and controlling the stress in your life before going to testosterone therapy. Get rid of excess body fat, especially your belly, since this elevates your estrogen levels and pushes testosterone levels down. Make sure, however, that you don't lose body fat too fast (more than two pounds per week), because if your body thinks you are starving, testosterone levels will plummet and your muscles will shrink.

If all of these efforts fail to restore your healthy levels of testosterone, find a knowledgeable doctor who will help you. I must emphasize that a skilled, experienced practitioner who monitors blood testosterone levels and performs digital rectal exams along with PSA tests to screen for prostate cancer must administer your therapy. In my office, every man undergoes a highly comprehensive evaluation to first determine if a clinical hormone deficiency exists. Any man needing a correction of hormone deficiencies has blood work done at six weeks, and again every three to four months after that to ensure that levels stay in the healthy range.

Because every man's hormone level is unique to him, it's impossible to know exactly how high your levels were before they declined. For this reason, most men require some fine-tuning of their treatments until the best results are achieved. You should notice that your symptoms begin to improve in three to six weeks after you start treatment.

Not every man is a good candidate for testosterone therapy. Discuss your current health status with your doctor, especially if you have a history of obstructive sleep apnea or heart failure. If you have one of these you need to see an appropriate specialist before starting therapy.

CHAPTER 11

The Growth Hormone Controversy

Human growth hormone (hGH) has been the subject of magazine covers, federal investigations, and television exposés. It has been abused by sports figures and celebrities as well as adamantly dismissed by many conventional physicians. And yet, research tells a different story: When hGH is correctly used, it has been clinically proven to improve health in men who have a documented clinical deficiency.

I have strong feelings about human growth hormone therapies because I have witnessed remarkable reversals in aging and disease by using it myself. I also want to make it very clear that like any type of medicine, it should not be abused, and it should be used only when it is determined to be absolutely necessary. This chapter is meant to give you all the information you need to help you decide with your doctor if growth hormone therapy is right for you.

The Backstory

The practice of age management medicine began in the 1990s when Dr. Daniel Rudman published a landmark article in the *New England Journal of Medicine.* Dr. Rudman looked at the effects of supplementing growth hormone in healthy men between the ages of 61 and 81. In this group of 21 men, Dr. Rudman managed to increase their lean muscle by 8.8 percent, decrease their fat mass by 14.4 percent, increase their skin thickness by 7 percent, and increase lumbar bone density by 1.6 percent, simply by giving injections of human growth hormone three times a week over a six-month period. The results of Dr. Rudman's study were confirmed and even extended in a study recently completed by the National Institute on Aging and Johns Hopkins University, headed by Doctors Mark Blackman and Mitch Harmon. Similar findings have been demonstrated with several other studies.

Since then, age management medicine physicians have embraced growth hormone as a treatment option for adults. Previously, it was used to extend growth for children. Until 1986 human growth hormone was harvested from cadavers and carried a risk for transmission of disease to its recipients. Since 1986, however, growth hormone has been commercially produced in the laboratory and the problem of disease transmission is no longer applicable. Today the supply of hGH is safe, available, and easy to administer. Unfortunately, hGH is expensive, though the costs of treating the diseases associated with untreated growth hormone deficiency over your lifetime far outweigh this expense.

Just as with unregulated testosterone use, we know that some athletes abuse this treatment when they take hGH to increase strength and improve their performance. It's important to know that hGH treatments are completely legal if you're diagnosed as being deficient and an FDA-approved formulation is obtained with a doctor's prescription after appropriate clinical testing proves your deficiency.

Another myth that has captured public attention is that growth hormone replacement therapy may put individuals at increased risk for developing a cancerous malignancy. The literature, however, does not support this notion. Current clinical guidelines from the Endocrine Society state that there is no evidence that the incidence of tumors is increased by growth hormone therapy. In 2001, the Growth Hormone Research Society extensively reviewed the question of whether growth hormone therapy is associated with tumor growth. Their final statement was quite telling: For patients receiving growth hormone therapy, "No additional monitoring for other malignant tumors (such as tumors of the prostate, breast, or colon) is currently suggested beyond the accepted standard of care for the patient's age and sex."

Signs and Symptoms of Growth Hormone Deficiency

Human growth hormone is naturally produced by the pituitary gland in your brain and is critical for repair throughout your body. Its ability to reverse many of the major effects of aging, including muscle loss, weakness, skin tone and texture, excess body fat deposits, energy depletion, and declining immune function, is unparalleled in today's medicine. It can also help boost your sex drive as well as sexual potency.

As we age, our growth hormone production decreases. Adult hGH levels decline by half from age 20 to age 60, and the loss accelerates thereafter. The following are some of the signs that you may be experiencing a decline of growth hormone:

- Decreased energy and vitality

- Decreased libido

- Decreased muscular strength

- Depression

- Diabetes

- Dyslipidemia

- Endothelial dysfunction

- Fatigue

- Hypertension

- Hypothyroidism

- Memory loss

- Metabolic Syndrome

- Obesity

- Osteoporosis

- Poor cognitive stability

- Reduced exercise capacity

- Sarcopenia

- Sleep apnea

- Sleep disturbance

How Growth Hormone Works

Growth hormone is a protein-based polypeptide hormone. It stimulates growth, cell reproduction, and regeneration in humans. Somatotropin refers to the growth hormone produced naturally in humans, whereas the term somatropin refers to growth hormone created by recombinant DNA technology and is abbreviated "hGH." Mounting evidence shows that adults with a somatotropin deficiency have impaired health, which then improves with hGH replacement therapy. When prescribed and monitored properly, this treatment is very safe and has the potential to greatly improve quality of life and reduce the incidence of morbidities associated with untreated growth hormone deficiency.

The following are diseases related to growth hormone deficiency:

- **Cardiovascular disease:** Growth hormone protects against endothelial dysfunction, atherosclerotic plaque development, Metabolic Syndrome, plaque instability, and ischemic myocardial damage. Low levels may represent an additional independent risk factor for cardiovascular disease.

- **Stroke:** Low levels of circulating growth hormone may be a predictor of stroke.

- **Obesity:** The health risks associated with obesity are closely correlated with abdominal, or visceral fat. Visceral fat causes Metabolic Syndrome, which is associated with serious metabolic disorders, including silent inflammation, heart disease, cancer, stroke, insulin resistance, diabetes, and Alzheimer's disease. Visceral fat is associated with a decrease in normal growth hormone levels. Numerous studies of growth hormone replacement therapy have found that treatment decreases fat mass and increases lean body mass.

Testing for a Deficiency

Doctors like me who administer growth hormone must adhere to federal guidelines. First, every doctor must conduct the appropriate testing required before administering this treatment to make sure that there is a clinical deficiency. The gold standard for diagnosing a growth hormone deficiency has been the insulin tolerance test (ITT): It has been the stimulation test used the most by endocrinologists. Another stimulation test is the glucagon stimulation test, which is considered much safer than the ITT. Many investigators and clinicians reject the ITT and other stimulation tests for diagnosing adult growth hormone deficiency and rely on a blood test called IGF-1 as a more reliable diagnostic and therapeutic marker of growth hormone deficiency.

In spite of all this controversy over the best method of diagnosing adult growth hormone deficiency, the FDA and hGH manufacturers have maintained their positions that stimulation testing is necessary and required for an accurate diagnosis. In my practice, I use glucagon pituitary stimulation testing as a prerequisite for diagnosing growth hormone deficiency.

I believe that before any man starts growth hormone therapy, he should be given an opportunity to improve his own production of growth hormone through correction of other hormone deficiencies and following a comprehensive program, such as the Life Plan, that maximizes diet and requires significant exercise. This strategy should be followed for at least six to eight weeks. After that, if growth hormone levels remain low and the signs and symptoms have not improved, I will consider performing a stimulation test to confirm my suspicions of growth hormone deficiency. Once therapy begins, all of my patients receiving hGH must be followed closely with repeat blood draws every three to four months to ensure that their levels are in the correct range and markers of disease are improving.

SKIP hGH THERAPY IF YOU HAVE

1. Pituitary stimulation testing not performed, or if performed, you passed the test and are not hGH deficient

2. A cancerous malignancy

3. Past history of malignancy (with the exception of basal cell carcinoma)

4. Diabetic proliferative retinopathy

5. Sclerosing diseases of the liver or lungs

6. Benign intracranial hypertension

7. Uncontrolled diabetes

Improve Your Production of Natural Growth Hormone

If you are clinically growth hormone deficient—and even if you aren't—you can retrain your brain to create more of this important hormone by taking better care of your health. Proper exercise and better nutrition can increase your production of growth hormone. I'm pleased when my patients follow my Life Plan protocol, because typically these men are able to come back to my office after just eight weeks with significant increases in their growth hormone levels. Once the body learns to do this, it will continue increased production as you continue the program.

Exercise can play a significant role in growth hormone secretion. About 10 to 20 minutes of aerobic exercise causes a rise in serum level that peaks at the end of that period and is sustained for up to two hours. If you train at 85 percent or more of your target HR_{max} for 20 to 25 minutes, you will stimulate your pituitary gland to produce more growth hormone. The same applies to exercises in which you lift heavy weights, such as squats, dead lifts, and bench presses, that involve large muscle groups.

If you were looking for the proverbial "last straw" in order to stop bad eating habits, it's well documented that a high-saturated-fat, low-carbohydrate diet reduces growth hormone secretion by 30 percent. On the other hand, following a diet high in protein and healthy fat increases your levels. Amino acids such as arginine, found in all protein sources, stimulate growth hormone secretion. Positive correlations have also been shown between growth hormone production and the intake of micronutrients such as calcium, iron, potassium, magnesium, niacin, phosphorus, riboflavin, thiamine, and zinc found in vegetables, fruits, and nutraceuticals. While the Life Healthy Eating Plan was initially developed for heart health, the growth hormone benefits are equally important.

We produce growth hormone all day long, but mostly during deep sleep. Men who don't sleep well or don't sleep enough will invariably have low levels of growth hormone, and many will be growth hormone deficient. This is one more reason that getting proper sleep is absolutely a must while you are following the Life Plan.

Mike Used the Life Plan to Restore His Growth Hormone

Mike was a 60-year-old accountant with a long history of weight problems when he first came to see me. Stuck in front of a computer most of the day, Mike was fairly inactive, and he had the gut to show for it: a 41-inch waist and 31.8 percent body fat. But that was just the beginning of Mike's problems: A bone density test in my office revealed he had osteoporosis.

I had Mike follow the Life Plan, beginning with the Basic Health Diet. I also started him on a weight-bearing workout at his gym, as well as vitamin D3 and calcium. I also restored his testosterone to healthy levels. After just one year, Mike no longer had osteoporosis. Instead, his bone density actually increased one standard deviation. He also was winning the battle of the bulge: His body fat dropped to 26.7 percent, and he lost 20 pounds. And he increased his IGF-1 into the low 200s from 88 without taking growth hormone.

CHAPTER 12

The Importance of Nutraceuticals

- -

The regular use of multivitamins and a few select nutritional supplements can measurably improve your nutritional status and lifelong health. Regardless of how healthy we eat, supplementing with quality nutraceuticals is critical, especially for men. Soils have long been depleted of vitamins and minerals from years of overfarming, chemical toxins, and acid rain. Supplementing your diet with key nutrients gives you the right vitamins, minerals, essential fatty acids, and antioxidants to optimize health, fight disease, improve libido, sharpen the mind, stabilize blood sugar/insulin, and maintain energy levels so that you can work out effectively and still have plenty of power for the rest of the day.

The truth is that most men do not consume sufficient amounts of the many nutrients we need from the foods we eat, even if we follow a careful diet, such as the Life Plan. Several years ago scientists thought that supplementing with vitamins and minerals was necessary only to prevent such diseases as scurvy, pellagra, and rickets—diseases we rarely hear about today. Now nutritional experts are beginning to understand that these types of micronutrients play key roles in the prevention of heart disease, cancer, arthritis, and cataracts, along with the signs and symptoms of aging, including loss of muscle mass, strength, and bone mass.

Men who push their bodies hard with aerobic and resistance training exercises, like those I have described in my Life Plan Workouts, definitely need additional nutritional support. During exercise, your sweat is detoxing your system, and as you lose water, you are also losing essential nutrients. We also require increased amounts of both macronutrients (carbohydrates, fats, and proteins) and micronutrients (vitamins and minerals) to make sure our metabolic machinery runs at peak performance to support our workouts.

The Oxidative Stress Factor

Oxidative stress is another very important reason active men need to make sure that they are getting the right amount of micronutrients. Oxidative stress occurs as a direct result of the additional oxygen required during exercise to carry out all of the desirable fat-burning and muscle-building reactions we work hard to activate.

This extra oxygen can act as a double-edged sword. It not only provides the essential ingredient that enables us to create a lean, muscular, healthy body, it also produces dangerous free radicals. Free radicals are the electronically unstable oxygen molecules that must scavenge electrons from whatever sources they can to become stable molecules. The sources of electrons can include DNA, cell membranes, important enzymes, and vital structural or functional proteins. When these important cell parts and substances lose their electrons to these free radicals, their function is altered, and the results can be catastrophic—cancer, heart disease, dementia, arthritis, muscle damage, increased susceptibility to infection, and accelerated aging. Worse, even though the Life Plan is making you healthier, it is working against you in terms of free radicals: Working out at 80 percent or more of your predicted HR_{max} for at least five hours per week can greatly increase the risk of your body tissues' suffering from excess free radicals.

VITAMINS AND CANCER RISK

The National Foundation for Cancer Research says an inadequate intake of essential micronutrients may increase the risk for cancer. Their scientific data indicate that nutritional factors may contribute to up to 60 percent of all cancer cases in the world, and are related to almost one-third of all cancer deaths in the United States each year.

The good news is that the fix is relatively easy. Antioxidants found in colorful fruits and vegetables can help protect us from these free radicals. However, most authorities believe that active men need far more than can be obtained from these natural sources, unless you are willing to sit down to a gallon of blueberries every morning. Supplementation with relatively high doses of the known antioxidants, which include vitamins C, E, and A, the mineral selenium, and phytochemicals, is probably the most reasonable way to address this issue. Antioxidants will not only help prevent the degenerative diseases I described above, they will also speed up your recovery from high-intensity workouts, promote muscle and strength building, and prevent exercise-related muscle injuries.

The Life Plan Nutraceutical Shopping List

Here's my list of the most important nutraceuticals I believe every active man needs in order to optimize his health and quality of life. Remember, more is not always better. Take these supplements as I've directed, and talk to your doctor about them as well. Also, it's best to split your daily supplements into a morning dose and an evening dose, because this allows your body to maintain a sufficient level of the water-soluble antioxidants needed to fight off free radicals. It really doesn't matter which ones you take when. Most comprehensive multivitamins/minerals are packaged in such a way that you take one serving in the morning and the other in the

THE DIFFERENCE BETWEEN VITAMINS AND MINERALS

Vitamins are organic compounds required as a nutrient in small amounts. Minerals, on the other hand, are elements that originate in earth and cannot be made by living organisms.

evening. I divide my fish oil into a morning serving and an evening serving. Melatonin should be taken at night because it enhances sleep. Some of my patients think vitamin D3 also helps them achieve a more restful sleep. As you read through the details for each of these supplement suggestions, you'll also see how they work together, and which should be taken at the same time.

The following is the basic nutraceutical shopping list. You can adapt this based on your current health and your own doctor's recommendations. On the Life Plan, I suggest that you take:

1. Comprehensive multivitamin and mineral supplement

2. Essential fatty acids

3. Probiotic supplement

4. Vitamin D3

5. CoQ 10

6. Saw palmetto

7. Lycopene

8. Milk thistle

9. Calcium

10. Pycnogenol/L-arginine

Comprehensive Multivitamin and Mineral Supplement

Every man needs a good multivitamin and mineral supplement every day. Use of a multivitamin/mineral formula can increase micronutrient profiles up to 35 percent. Make sure you pick one that has at least 100 percent of the Recommended Dietary Allowance (RDA) for thiamin (B1), riboflavin (B2), niacin (B3), vitamins B6, B12, E, and folic acid. You also need 2,000 milligrams of vitamin C, at least 400 IU of vitamin E, and at least 100 milligrams of magnesium. Your multivitamin should also contain at least 20 micrograms of vitamin K, as well as the minerals chromium, copper, selenium, and zinc (15 mg). If you are on a blood thinner (such as Coumadin), talk with your doctor about how much vitamin K you require.

Read labels carefully for the amount of vitamin A you should take. Too much can lead to toxicity and bone loss. Vitamin A toxicity can easily be avoided by simply taking beta-carotene, which your body converts to vitamin A. The vitamin A in supplements can come from retinol (often called vitamin A palmitate or acetate). To protect your bones, limit retinol to no more than 3,000 IU per day. Less is better. Beta-carotene doesn't cause bone loss, but too much beta-carotene may increase the risk of lung cancer if you are a smoker (which you shouldn't be, but you know that already). You don't need more than 15,000 IU daily of beta-carotene.

Essential Fatty Acids (Fish Oil Supplements)

Omega-3 and omega-6 fatty acids are essential fatty acids that we cannot make in our bodies and must, therefore, consume from food sources or supplements. Americans consume roughly 10 times more omega-6 fatty acids than omega-3 fatty acids. These large amounts of omega-6 fatty acids typically come from vegetable oils containing linoleic acid (corn oil, safflower oil, sesame oil) and produce an unhealthy imbalance in the omega-3 to omega-6 fatty acid ratio, which contributes to heart and blood vessel disease.

To strike a better balance, we need to increase our consumption of omega-3 fatty acid. This is typically found in cold-water, fatty fish such as salmon, striped sea bass, tuna (albacore), sardines, herring, mackerel, and whitefish. The American Heart Association recommends a minimum intake of two fish meals weekly for primary cardiovascular protection. This is difficult for many men to achieve because suitable fish are increasingly expensive and hard to find. The supply of wild salmon and other species that are not contaminated with mercury and other pollutants is increasingly restricted. An alternative is to take dietary supplements rich in DHA/EPA in the form of high-quality fish oil capsules that have had mercury and other pollutants removed.

Fish oil fatty acids have anti-inflammatory effects and are helpful for combating inflammatory diseases such as rheumatoid arthritis. They are also considered protective against heart disease. To get the most healthful benefits, purchase high-quality fish oil supplements that have the highest amount of eicosapentaenoic acid, EPA, and docosahexaenoic acid, DHA, per capsule, and keep them refrigerated. You need to take four one-gram capsules daily in order to create the best balance for your body.

When looking for a high-quality product,

FOLATE IS ESSENTIAL FOR MUSCLE BUILDING

Folate, better known as folic acid, is one of the B vitamins that is necessary for the healthy division of cells and the prevention of colon cancer. It can also play a key role in the growth of new muscle tissue that is essential to increasing muscle mass and strength.

Folate also helps prevent heart and blood vessel disease by keeping homocystine levels low. Homocystine is a chemical our bodies produce that damages the linings of blood vessels, which starts the cascade of events that ultimately lead to a heart attack. Folate, along with the help of vitamins B6 and B12, converts homocystine into other harmless amino acids. A large government study in 2002 found that people who consumed the most folate had the fewest strokes and the least heart disease.

Poor diet and a heavy consumption of alcohol work together to drastically lower natural folate levels. The best way to make sure you are getting enough folate is to eat plenty of green vegetables, beans, some fruits, and wheat germ. Or, make sure your multivitamin contains 400 micrograms of this essential vitamin.

always read the list of ingredients found on the bottle. If additives or preservatives have been added to increase shelf life, they might make the overall supplement less effective. Ultrarefined and ultrapurified fish oil products are better choices. These companies are using pharmaceutical-grade fish oil in their supplement processing. In addition to this, the content of high-quality fish oil should be made up of at least 60 percent of both essential fatty acids (EPA and DHA) combined. The concentration of DHA should not be less than 18 percent, and a higher concentration

VITAMIN E

Because fish oil does not contain enough fat-soluble antioxidants to compensate for potential oxidative damage, it's also a good idea to increase your intake of vitamin E as you increase your fish oil consumption. Between 400 and 800 IU of vitamin E per day, in the form of mixed tocopherols, should cover this increase. Although fish oil capsules and your multivitamin also contain some vitamin E, it may not be enough.

is a signal of superior quality. Overall, DHA is more important for our body than EPA and helps in fighting against many diseases.

Buy only products that have undergone molecular distillation. Molecular distillation not only removes the impurities found in fish oil in the form of mercury and dioxins, but also balances out the concentration of other nutrients, such as vitamin A and D, if present. So, high-quality fish oil is processed and packed after going through the process of molecular or high-vacuum distillation.

Finally, you should be able to determine from the packaging what type of fish the oil comes from, and where the fish was actually caught. The highest-quality fish oil supplements are made in New Zealand and Norway. Oily fish found in these regions of the world are less contaminated, and the oil obtained from them does not require as much purification.

If you take cod liver oil (a few men prefer this to fish oil capsules), be aware that it also contains vitamins A and D. Depending on how much cod liver oil you use and what other supplements you're taking, you could be getting too much of these vitamins. An alternative is devitaminized cod liver oil.

Probiotic Supplement

Probiotics are live microorganisms (in most cases, bacteria) that are similar to the beneficial microorganisms normally found in the human gut. They are also referred to as "friendly bacteria" or "good bacteria." Probiotics are not the same as prebiotics, which are nondigestible food ingredients that selectively stimulate the growth or activity of beneficial microorganisms already in the colon. Probiotics may help with a number of health problems, according to the National Center for Complementary and Alternative Medicine (NCCAM) and the American Society for Microbiology. These include gastrointestinal distress, symptoms of lactose intolerance, inflammation reduction, cancer prevention, and enhanced micronutrient absorption.

Probiotics are available in foods and dietary supplements. Food sources include unpasteurized yogurt (which is difficult to find), fermented and unfermented milk, miso, tempeh, and some juices. Dietary supplements are available in the form of capsules, powders, and tablets. Dosages are listed by organism quantity—in "billions of organisms."

There has recently been strong interest among the sporting community in the potential benefits of probiotics in reducing susceptibility to upper respiratory infections and gastrointestinal illness. Studies are under way to confirm the mechanisms by which probiotics enhance immunity. In the meantime, I think it is prudent to include probiotics in your nutraceutical regimen. Choose one that is a blend of at least six "live" cultures that is kept in a refrigerated case, and make sure to keep it refrigerated at home. Follow the manufacturer's recommended dosing on the label, since dosage can differ depending on the probiotic source.

Vitamin D3

Vitamin D is really a form of steroid hormone, not a vitamin. Adequate vitamin D levels protect people against cancer, heart disease, infections, premature aging, all age-related diseases, and death. A June 2008 study reported that vitamin D deficiency gives men a 2.5 times higher risk for a heart attack. They also found that men with intermediate vitamin D levels demonstrated a 60 percent increased myocardial infarction risk. Vitamin D is also essential for the proper absorption of calcium, which is why it is critical that every man gets enough to promote bone growth and prevent osteoporosis.

Most men who work indoors have insufficient or deficient levels of vitamin D. Eating vitamin D–rich foods cannot solve the problem alone. Vitamin D is mostly (90 percent) manufactured in our skin when we are exposed to sunlight. During the winter months the sun's rays are just not strong enough in the northern climates to promote vitamin D synthesis. If you live in the northern third of the United States, Canada, or Alaska, you're probably not getting enough vitamin D during the winter months. This, combined with the fact that most winter activity is limited to the indoors, results in very little sun exposure.

A blood test for 25-hydroxy-vitamin D is the best way to determine your status. Levels less than 30 ng/ml are considered to be a deficiency state. Optimal levels are 60 to 90 ng/ml. Most of my patients need to take 5,000 IU to 10,000 IU daily to achieve these levels, which is significantly more than what is offered in even the best multivitamin. Make sure to talk to your doctor about vitamin D supplementation if you are currently taking antiseizure medications.

Coenzyme Q$_{10}$

Coenzyme Q$_{10}$ is a vitamin-like chemical that is found in practically all the cells in the body, especially the heart. It has antioxidant properties, and the body uses it to generate ATP, the cellular storage unit of energy. Coenzyme Q$_{10}$ levels start declining after the age of 20. A low level of CoQ$_{10}$ is thought to interfere with energy production pathways in our body.

The potential benefits of taking CoQ$_{10}$ include antioxidant activity, prevention of age-related macular degeneration, enhancing athletic performance, improved immune function, prevention of heart disease, and slowing the aging process. Any man who is taking a statin drug to control cholesterol levels must take extra coenzyme Q$_{10}$ because statins deplete CoQ$_{10}$ from skeletal and cardiac muscle. The recommended dose of coenzyme Q$_{10}$ is 100 milligrams if you are not on a statin and 200 milligrams daily if you are on a statin.

Saw Palmetto

Saw palmetto is used mainly for relieving urinary symptoms associated with an enlarged prostate gland (benign prostatic hyperplasia, or BPH), such as frequent nighttime urination. Several small studies suggest that saw palmetto may be effective for treating BPH symptoms. However, a 2009 review of the research concluded that saw palmetto has not been shown to be more effective than a placebo for this use.

My experience is mixed. Some of my patients, as well as I, believe it has significantly helped reduce the frequency and number of times they have to get up at night. Others feel it hasn't helped them much. I think it's worthwhile to give it a try, since it is well tolerated by most men. Look for a supplement that is standardized to contain 85 to 95 percent fatty acids and sterols. The recommended dose is 160 milligrams twice a day.

Lycopene

Lycopene is a phytochemical that creates the bright red pigment found in tomatoes and other red fruits and vegetables, such as watermelons and papayas (but not strawberries or cherries). Lycopene is an antioxidant that has been considered a potential agent for prevention of some types of cancers, particularly prostate cancer, because preliminary research has shown an inverse correlation between consumption of tomatoes and cancer risk.

I think it is prudent to take 20 milligrams daily of this nutrient to err on the safe side of nutritional health. Compare this dosage to the ingredients in your multivitamin to ensure that you are covered: Many multis include lycopene. It is better absorbed when taken with a fatty acid, so make sure to take it at the same time as your fish oil supplements.

Milk Thistle

The seeds of the milk thistle have been used for over 2,000 years to treat chronic liver disease and protect the liver against toxins. Increasing research is being undertaken on the physiological effects, therapeutic properties, and possible medical uses of milk thistle. In a 2009 study of 50 children, published in the journal *Cancer*, milk thistle showed promise in reducing the liver-damaging effects of chemotherapy.

The literature supports the benefits of milk thistle in protecting the liver, and I would encourage all men to take this supplement. Look for a standardized extract that contains 70 percent silymarin at the dose of 200 milligrams twice a day.

Calcium

Calcium is the most abundant mineral in the body. It is naturally found in some foods and is added to others, such as milk products. It is also available as a dietary supplement and is present in most antacids. Calcium is required for muscle contraction, blood vessel expansion and contraction, secretion of hormones and enzymes, and transmitting impulses throughout the nervous system. The body strives to maintain constant concentrations of calcium in blood, muscle, and intercellular fluids. When our intake of calcium is low, our bodies resort to pulling calcium from our bones to maintain these critical concentrations. Then, as we age, our weakened bones break down from calcium loss, resulting in bone density loss that increases the risk of osteoporosis. Men need calcium supplementation as much as women. I frequently see men in my practice who have early or full-blown osteoporosis.

Calcium requires its own set of pills, because you need 1,000 to 1,200 milligrams daily, which is far less than what is available in a typical multivitamin. The two main forms of calcium found in supplements are calcium carbonate and calcium citrate. Calcium carbonate is more commonly available and is both inexpensive and convenient. Both the carbonate and citrate forms are similarly well absorbed, but men taking medications such as Pepcid that reduce levels of stomach acid can absorb calcium citrate more easily.

LARRY L. LEWIN

"In October 2009 I was 58 years old weighing over 215 pounds. I had just suffered the third kidney stone attack in five years, my EKG results were very poor, and I had an operation on a deviated septum. As a person who had been healthy all of his life, I came to realize that if I did not change my quality of life going forward it would change for me. As one would say, fate had something to do with me getting the chance to work with Dr. Life.

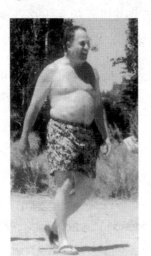

"I received a promotional postcard in the mail and my wife called to set up an appointment. October 2009 was the beginning of the second half of my life. After meeting the team, understanding the program, taking the required vitamins and nutrients, while at the same time adjusting my diet, I have been able to make great personal strides. Just a year later I weighed in at 196½ pounds. My body fat count went from 39 percent to 33 percent, and all my blood work has shown great improvement."

Pycnogenol Plus L-arginine

Great sex requires a strong erection, which relies on the relaxation of the cavernous smooth muscle and dilation of blood vessels, which are triggered by the chemical nitric oxide (NO). Pycnogenol, a natural plant extract from the bark of the maritime pine tree, increases the production of your own nitric oxide. When Pycnogenol is combined with L-arginine, the supplement formed has been shown to produce a significant improvement in sexual function in men with erectile dysfunction, without any side effects. The best dose is 40 milligrams of Pycnogenol, two times a day, and 2 grams of L-arginine once a day. I have personally used this combination of supplements and can attest to its effectiveness for men with or without erectile dysfunction.

Choosing a Reliable Resource for Supplements

One common complaint about supplements is that they are sold in a completely unregulated market. It is very difficult to know exactly what you are buying, especially if you are shopping at a drugstore or health-food store. Your goal should be purchasing supplements of the highest quality, which generally means buying the more expensive brands. Shop at a store with a good reputation that can give you good advice about the quality of their products. Checking out products online is another good idea. Remember that capsules are generally more readily absorbed into your body than tablets.

There are several excellent quality vitamin and mineral supplements available on the market. Cenegenics nutraceuticals are high-quality, pharmaceutical-grade products that I recommend. Dr. Kenneth H. Cooper has also created a line of excellent vitamin and mineral supplements. These products can be reviewed on his website, www.coopercomplete.com.

IT'S NOT ENOUGH JUST TO BUY THEM, YOU HAVE TO TAKE YOUR SUPPLEMENTS

The most important rule about supplements is taking them consistently. They cannot help you if you let them sit in your cabinet. It sometimes takes several weeks to feel the effects or to notice them working, but continue to take them to maximize your results.

Vitamin and mineral supplementation alone won't get you all the thousands of micronutrients that are responsible for a multitude of health benefits. Even the best supplementation program must work with a balanced diet, such as the ones I created for the Life Plan. This is why you need to make sure you eat plenty of nontropical fruits, vegetables, healthy fats, and high-quality, lean protein.

One of his products is called Cooper Complete Elite Athlete formulation. This is a vitamin/mineral supplement designed specifically for high-endurance aerobic athletes, but I believe that it works equally well for anyone involved in high-intensity resistance training. It does lack calcium, so be sure you add a 1,000- or 1,200-milligram supplement to your regimen if you take this product.

Another great source of high-quality supplements is Nutrascriptives. For more information on all of these supplements, check out my website, www.drlife.com.

CHAPTER 13

The Life Plan for the Future: Breakthrough Medicine

Y ou now have a much better understanding of what it takes to become sexier, stronger, and leaner. No matter your age, you can begin the Life Plan knowing that you are doing the very best for your body now, and for your future health. I hope that you find this program to be as rewarding as I have. There is no way that I could have made this transformation without it. I know that if I can change from being a fat old man to becoming a healthier, leaner, and in all respects younger man, you can, too.

Doing the work is completely up to you. But I can tell you that the more time and effort you put in, the better the results will be. Best of all, you can continue to follow this program for the rest of your life without making too many adjustments. I can't tell you how many men I've seen revert to their old ways and, consequently, their old bodies. That's not going to be in my future, and it shouldn't be in yours. And that's certainly not what healthy-aging doctors like me mean by "turning back the clock."

Now, let's take a real look forward into what's next in age management medicine. The three hottest topics right now are genetic testing, stem cell banking, and telomeres. I am fortunate to be involved with the cutting edge of all of these medical breakthroughs.

Genetic Testing: You Can Control Your Future Health

Today's medical technology allows each of us to begin to take a proactive stance on future health. Preventive medicine is more than consistent diet and exercise; it's about testing your health earlier, and often. Genetic testing can be a smart preventive step to detecting your propensity for certain conditions.

Chromosomes form your genetic material, called the genome. Each of your cells has 23 pairs of chromosomes, with each half inherited from your mother and father. These structures have extremely long, double-stranded DNA—nuclear DNA—made up of subunits called "genes." Your genotype is determined by your cell's unique gene combination. These aren't the observable, physical traits (height, hair color, eye color, skin tone), but rather internal genetic variations that cause you to be unique.

Genetic testing enables doctors to analyze your genetic makeup in order to diagnose a medical condition or your risk of or vulnerabilities to inherited diseases. Clinicians isolate mutations or alterations in your genetic code that are associated with genetic disorders. Testing these mutations can help diagnose (or rule out) a possible genetic condition, or determine your risk of developing certain diseases in the future. It can even tell us whether your family members are at risk for the same disorder.

Diagnosing Current Disease

Diagnostic genetic testing can be performed at any time throughout your life. It can be performed on a variety of types of diseases, including infectious disease. Bacteria, viruses, and parasites have their own genetic code, and genetic testing can be used to uncover them. Genetic testing is also useful in determining how well a therapy is combating infections such as HIV and hepatitis C.

Some examples of genetically associated diseases that typically affect men are:

- Alzheimer's disease

- Bone marrow disorders

- Cardiovascular disease

- Celiac disease

- Colon cancer

- Cystic fibrosis

- Diabetes

- Down syndrome

- Leukemia

- Lupus

- Lymphoma

- Obesity

- Osteoarthritis

- Sickle-cell disease

Predicting Future Disease

Several methods are available for testing genetic predisposition or risk of future disease. This type of genetic testing can help identify mutations that could lead to genetic-associated disorders before any signs or symptoms appear, and can be performed at any life stage. Knowing what the future might hold is one important step you need to take to be able to make informed decisions about your healthcare.

For the results to be meaningful, more than one type of test may be necessary, and your family members may need to be tested. A genetic consultation can help determine what tests are needed and who should be tested as well as explain costs and what can be gleaned from the results.

There are over 1,200 genetic tests available, with even more on the way. Here is a sampling of the most popular types among researchers and forward-thinking doctors:

Direct testing—Direct examination of DNA/RNA within the gene.

Indirect/linkage testing—Search for markers that are associated with a disease-causing gene.

Biochemical testing—Analysis of metabolites and enzymes to look for errors of metabolism that can lead to disease.

Cytogenetic testing—Evaluation of the number and shape of chromosomes for signs of abnormality.

Testing Procedures

- -

Your primary physician, genetics specialist/counselor, or nurse practitioner can order the necessary testing. A sample of genetic material—blood, urine, saliva, stool, body tissue, bone, or hair—is taken and shipped to a laboratory. The genetic material then undergoes extractions. Cells are broken apart, and the genes are isolated and later manipulated and evaluated.

Your results may not present black-and-white answers. As with other medical tests, there is room for interpretation. Equally important is what you choose to do with the information, and how to structure the rest of your life based on the results of the testing.

ARE GENETIC SERVICES FOR ME?

If you are Afro-American, Asian, East Indian, French-Canadian, Greek, Italian, or Jewish, there are special genetic testing methods available. If you have a family history of birth defects, Alzheimer's, autoimmune diseases, blindness, sickle-cell trait, Down syndrome, colon cancer, early onset cancer/emphysema/heart disease (under 35), mental retardation, muscular dystrophy, or hemophilia, you are also a candidate for genetic testing. And if you have a personal medical history of diabetes, cancer, degenerative diseases, hearing loss, blindness, mental illness, or seizures, you may be able to learn more about your future health through genetic testing.

The Next Step: Gene Therapy

- -

Researchers are currently working with genes and learning how to correct disabling or fatal diseases triggered by a gene deficiency or gene abnormality. Studies are under way investigating whether gene therapy can treat heart disease, AIDS, or even cancer. Admittedly experimental, gene therapy holds promise for the future.

This type of therapy could happen in various ways:

- Replacing a mutated gene with a healthy copy

- Deactivating a mutated gene

- Inserting a healthy gene to battle disease

Breakthrough Medicine: Adult Stem Cell Therapy

Adult stem cells are taken from your bone marrow and peripheral blood. No embryo is destroyed in collecting adult stem cells. Even though these are taken from a single location, stem cells are powerful master cells that can morph into a number of specialized cell types. The bone marrow cells can regenerate almost anywhere in the body where they are placed. Then they work by renewing immune cells, tissues, organs, and our blood. In general, stem cell therapies are referred to as *regenerative medicine.*

Stem cell therapies are on the cutting edge of medical breakthroughs, not only for their restorative properties fighting diseases, but for their general antiaging benefits. Currently, there are no therapies that have been approved for use by the FDA, although I believe that will change in the very near future. However, many American men currently travel to other countries around the world where these therapies are being developed.

There are several conditions being treated right now with adult stem cell therapy, including leukemias, lymphoma, multiple myeloma, coronary heart disease, radiation sickness, multiple sclerosis, lupus, autoimmune diseases, tissue repair/burns, type 1 diabetes and orthopedics, sickle cell, aplastic anemia, neurological disorders, and arthritis. Regenerative therapy also has a strong potential for treating spinal cord injuries, strokes, severe infectious diseases, Lou Gehrig's disease, type 2 diabetes, osteoporosis, autoimmune neurological diseases, and amyloidosis (abnormal protein buildup in tissues). Research has presented significant findings from over 2,000 FDA-funded clinical trials.

One of the most promising areas of interest is stem cell research and heart disease. Heart attacks destroy heart tissue and drain the heart's muscle cells. Scientists are learning how stem cells can be used to regenerate and activate new blood vessels. They are also finding that stem cells are showing clinical benefits for severe chronic heart disease (congestive heart failure).

In the United States, the conversation surrounding stem cells that is most likely to affect consumers is creating a storage or "banking" system. In terms of stem cells, this is more of a medical insurance policy for the future than a treatment protocol we can use today. It is widely thought that by collecting and banking adult stem cells, and then infusing them into the body every few years, we will be able to slow the aging process. Stem cell banking is completely legal in the United States.

Banking Adult Stem Cells

Once stem cell therapies are approved in this country, you will be able to access public cell banks. However, because each of us is completely different, you will have only a 20 to 50 percent chance of finding a match within the public pool. Because I strongly believe that stem cell therapies are the next wave of breakthrough medicine, I am suggesting to my patients that they consider banking their own stem cells after completing a few months of the Life Plan, when they are most healthy. Although adult stem cells can be harvested even into your 80s, healthier, younger cells are always the richest. And even more to the point, stem cell health is negatively affected by poor lifestyle choices and illness.

If you are interested in pursuing this, as you follow the Life Plan over the next few months, increase your intake of foods that are high in antioxidants, such as blueberries, tomatoes, and green tea. These foods, as well as vitamin D3, are known to increase bone marrow growth by 83 percent. Omega-3 fatty acids, including the fish oil supplements you will be taking, have been shown to help repair adult stem cells. Finally, hormone therapy has been shown to enhance stem cell effects, according to research with testosterone and growth hormone replacement.

Once collected, the stem cells are treated at a processing laboratory, then made ready

STEM CELL FACTS

- Two major types of stem cells exist: adult and embryonic.

- Adult stem cells are found naturally in the human body as well as in umbilical cord blood.

- Live adult stem cells are produced in bone marrow and circulate throughout the bloodstream, tissues, and organs.

- Adult stem cells can be harvested from anyone weighing 80 pounds or more. Better stem cell quality/potency comes from younger, healthier persons.

- Over 70 diseases have been treated successfully with adult stem cells.

- Banking your own is a smart move. It ensures a perfect match and quick availability whenever you need them; your body won't reject them.

- Families often bank together so they can share cells with each other.

for permanent cryogenic storage—a process that ensures cell integrity. Cooled to far below freezing, the adult stem cells enter a subfrozen state before being stored in a tank filled with liquid nitrogen (–196° C) where they can be kept for years. Stem cells can't be refrozen, so they are kept in a determined number of containers to be taken and thawed as needed.

Telomeres: The Future Is Now

Telomeres are DNA repeats located at the end of chromosomes that act as caps to protect genes. Telomeres shorten every time a cell divides, causing a cellular digression and conditions associated with aging, and eventually, death. In order to prevent the ravages of aging as we get older, we need to learn how to lengthen our telomeres now, or prevent the ones we have from getting any shorter. Short telomeres lead to premature cellular aging and an enhanced risk of cancer, and of fatal cancer in particular.

In January 2009, I entered the telomere revolution, becoming a consultant for TA Sciences in New York, the first company worldwide to offer a synthetic version of telomerase—a natural enzyme—that can help maintain telomere length. Their product, TA-65™, is a nutraceutical that prevents telomeres from shortening. TA-65 comes from extracts of the Chinese herb astragalus, which has been used for medicinal purposes for more than 1,000 years. I am one of just a handful of physicians in the United States licensed to offer TA-65™ to my patients. It's important for all men to know about this amazing nutrient, and be ready to talk to their physician about it when it becomes more widely available.

This brand-new formulation allows men the best opportunity to maintain their quality of life as they age, reducing risk for disease and maybe even extending their life span. I can offer TA-65 to all my healthy-aging patients and have a few patients who are taking TA-65, with great results. For example, Bill is a molecular geneticist and a 100-mile run enthusiast, completing more 100-mile runs in 1998 than anyone else in the world. He retired from running in 1999 and began to devote most of his time to his research company. But once he switched his focus, he found that he had little exercise, which led to a sharp decline in his health. In midyear 2007, Bill started taking TA-65™ and started training again. He finished the 2008 and 2009 Badwater events (the "toughest foot race on the planet"), going from a "back-of-the-pack runner" to the front. He attributes his success to TA-65.

Other companies are starting to form that will target the science of lengthening telomeres. A new company that seems to hold particular promise is Telomere Sciences. Their first nutritional supplement, Telomere Length Formula, targets all three major causes of telomere shortening: aging, oxidative stress, and inflammation.

For more information, visit www.maxlife.org/Telomeres for a comprehensive resource for telomere health.

My colleague Calvin B. Harley, Ph.D., released in 2010 the first scientific paper that demonstrated the benefits in humans of activating telomerase. These benefits include immune system rejuvenation and lengthening of critically short telomeres. He and his collaborators were the first to demonstrate that telomere length is specifically lost with age in normal dividing cells, and that this process is responsible for cellular aging.

We also know that you can naturally increase levels of telomerase activity, which can take care of cellular damage and in turn increase the length of telomeres. The best way to do this is, once again, to just follow the Life Plan. By decreasing stress, eating healthy, and exercising properly, you can prevent telomeres from shortening while you are giving your body all it needs to continue feeling and looking young.

CHAPTER 14

Share the Life Plan with Your Doctor

The best of preventive medicine is in your own hands. You have the ability to look and feel younger and better, stronger and sexier, right now. You don't have to wait for science to catch up with you: You are on the leading edge. My goal for you is to embrace this program so that everyone you love notices the differences in your health and the way you look every time you walk into a room. More important, I want you to feel good about yourself, now, and well into the future.

As with any other wellness plan, talk to your doctor before you start my program. Let him or her understand that you are interested in a heart-healthy lifestyle that is meant to increase metabolism, prevent disease, and slow aging. Together, you can beat the system and join the revolution of healthy aging. Working with your doctor as a team is one of the best motivators that you will ever have to stay on the program. Your doctor can keep you accountable for reaching your goals, and monitor your health along the way.

The best place to start is with your current physician. However, it's important to recognize that many primary care providers may feel threatened when you bring up such subjects as age management medicine, because they may not be knowledgeable about the practices I preach. Bring this book with you, and show your M.D. or D.O. the reference section and the dozens of studies that support my work. If he or she still blows you off, telling you that "aging is just part of the game of life," then you are getting a clear signal that it's time to find another doctor.

Dr. Life's Top 10 Questions to Ask Your M.D./D.O.

These 10 questions will be your medical shopping list. If you don't like the answers you receive, it may be time to find yourself a new doctor.

1. If costs and insurance were not an issue, what would you do as my doctor to improve my quality of life as I age and to reduce my risks for age-related disease?

2. What would you recommend for nutritional supplementation that will reduce my risks for disease and possibly extend my lifespan?

3. What are your thoughts about correcting any hormonal deficiencies I may have that may improve my quality of life and reduce my risk for age-related disease?

4. Do HMOs or insurance companies affect or influence your decisions on what medications, diagnostic tests, or referrals to specialists you make regarding my medical care?

5. If you or a member of your family had my condition, what would you do?

6. If your primary care physician refers you to a specialist, ask: Is this the specialist you would use if *you* had this same problem?

7. Is your compensation affected by your prescribing patterns, referral patterns, or the diagnostic tests you order?

8. If insurance or costs weren't an issue, what advice, treatment, or medical/lab tests would you recommend that might provide early warning signs of diseases I may be at risk for?

9. Are there any alternative or complementary medical therapies that might help my medical condition?

10. How much training and education have you had about the role nutrition and exercise play in overall health?

Shop for the Best Medical Care

The doctor who is going to be the most receptive to the Life Plan is typically not an endocrinologist, a specialist who is trained to diagnose problems by helping to restore the normal balance of hormones. Endocrinologists focus on health issues such as diabetes, thyroid diseases, metabolic disorders, osteoporosis, hypertension, cholesterol (lipid) disorders, lack of growth (short stature), and cancers of the endocrine glands. While you may be affected by one or more of these conditions, the place to start is with a primary care physician who is either an M.D. or a D.O. who is familiar with andropause and its related issues, including the treatment of hormone deficiencies. Your doctor should also be able to talk about the importance of exercise and nutrition in a deeper way than, "You need to exercise more and eat less in order to lose weight."

You can interview potential doctors on the phone before your office visit, or talk to their office manager or their staff. Search the internet to see if they maintain a website that shares their medical philosophy. You can also find out if they have recently published, which is a good sign that the doctors in question are current with the latest findings. I don't recommend the various websites that rate doctors: I find that these are often biased, or not always reliable.

You can also choose a doctor who is affiliated with a hospital that you would choose to be admitted to if you ever required serious hospitalization. However, many doctors like me who practice age management medicine are not affiliated with a hospital and are not considered "primary care physicians."

Most doctors you may consider are looking into this type of medicine as an addition to their current practice. Another option is a specialist in age management medicine like me. On my

DON'T WAIT FOR THE DOCTOR TO FIND A LIFE-THREATENING DISEASE

The next time you meet with your physician, tell the nurse checking you in that you want to talk about a specific issue, such as bone density. Once you bring up any health concern, it becomes what's known as a "chief complaint" and a permanent part of your medical record, making it incumbent upon the doctor to do something about it. So get the ball rolling and ask the right questions, weaving in any genetic factor potentials:

- "My parents died from age-related disease that started when they were relatively young. I'm here to do all I can to prevent or reverse age-related disease. Would you check my hormone levels, bone density, and cholesterol levels?"

- "My dad died in his 50s from heart disease. Don't you think I should get a calcium score . . . or perhaps a carotid artery ultrasound scan?"

website, www.drlife.com, is a listing of highly regarded age management medicine specialists across the country.

The Life Plan Standard of Care

In my office I exclusively practice age management medicine. Because my patients come from all over the country, I cannot always act as their primary care physician. Instead, I act as a resource—they talk to me about problems they have. If my patients need to be admitted to a hospital, I refer them back to their primary care provider or, when necessary, directly to a hospitalist, who is a physician who works exclusively within a hospital setting caring for hospitalized patients, as needed.

Men who come to my office for the very first time experience a thorough checkup, and I mean it. A typical first visit can last as long as seven hours. Before he comes in, each patient submits the blood work I have ordered, which includes 90 different tests, including hormone blood levels. In my office, each man then undergoes further diagnostic testing, including strength testing, ultrasound testing for blood vessel health, and a DEXA scan that measures body composition in terms of body fat and muscle mass. Then he meets with my exercise and nutrition specialist to develop a program that is specifically designed to meet his goals. After lunch I introduce the Life Plan. We then move to my office, where I discuss his goals, diagnostics, and lab work and create a blueprint for how he is going to modify his lifestyle for the best possible results based on his current health.

BRING THIS BOOK

Take the Life Plan with you to your annual checkup, and make sure to review with your doctor your list of personal goals that you are trying to achieve. Show the doctor your worksheets and journal entries to show him or her what you've already accomplished.

I know that many doctors are unable to provide this same level of care. Here is a list of the minimum requirements that your doctor should be providing in an annual checkup. Be prepared for an exam that should take at least sixty minutes. During this time, your visit should include:

1. The list of diagnostic testing (see list below).

2. A thorough physical exam, including a digital rectal exam of the prostate.

3. A detailed questionnaire, like the quiz in Chapter 1, that helps your physician detect early warning signs of premature aging or underlying illness.

Create a Baseline Health Record

The chart below lists all of the tests you should request as part of your routine medical care. These markers will help you take action early to prevent disease. What's more, they will create a wealth of baseline information that you can use to stay vital as you age and limit your exposure to "surprise" illnesses. These early warning tests can be used to prevent or delay their onset.

IMPORTANT TESTS TO MAINTAIN OPTIMAL HEALTH AND LOWER DISEASE RISK

Test	Definition	Optimal Results
Bone Density Test or DEXA Scan: Skeleton, Lumbar Spine, and Hips	This test determines whether you are at risk for osteoporosis, which causes bones to become fragile or break. A DEXA scan can also be used to monitor osteoporosis treatment as well as compute body composition (body fat percentage and muscle mass). The DEXA scan is a fast, painless, noninvasive procedure. It is not the same as a bone scan, which detects fractures, cancer, infections, and other abnormalities. Men over 45 should complete a DEXA scan annually.	T Score > 0
Complete Eye Exam (Glaucoma Testing and Amsler Grid)	This series of tests is designed to evaluate your vision and check for eye diseases. It is recommended that you have a complete exam every two to four years if you are between 40 and 65.	Negative
Blood Pressure	Blood pressure is the force exerted by circulation blood on the walls of blood vessels and is one of the principal vital signs. Maximum blood pressure is called systolic and minimum is diastolic. It is typically measured in millimeters of mercury.	120/80 or less

CANCER SCREENINGS

Test	Definition	Optimal Results
Colonoscopy	This test provides an inside look at your colon and rectum. Preparation for the test and the test itself are painless. If polyps (possible precancerous growths) are detected, they can be easily removed. This procedure is recommended for men starting at age 50 and should be repeated every 5 to 10 years. Men with a family history of polyps or certain cancers should consult their health professional to determine when to start and how often they should repeat their colonoscopies.	Negative
Digital Rectal Exam of Prostate	Used to screen for overall prostate health and prostate cancer in its early stages. This exam is done during a typical physical. It is recommended that African-American men and any man with a family history of prostate cancer begin having annual digital rectal exams at the age of 40. Caucasian men without a family history of prostate cancer should start at age 50.	Negative

Test	Definition	Optimal Results
Prostate Specific Antigen (PSA)	PSA is a protein produced by the cells of a prostate gland. This test measures the amount of PSA in the blood and is used primarily to screen for prostate cancer before symptoms occur. Prostate cancer, enlarged prostate, or prostate infections can increase the PSA level in men. This test is recommended starting at age 45, or in men at age 40 if they have a history of prostate cancer or are of African-American heritage.	0–3 ng/ml

BLOOD SUGAR CONTROL

Test	Definition	Optimal Results
Hemoglobin A1c (Glycohemoglobin)	This test provides a long-term look at blood sugar control and reflects the role nutrition, activity, medication, and stress play in blood sugar control. This test should be obtained 3 to 4 times a year.	<5.5%
Insulin (Fasting)	This test provides information about your body's sensitivity to insulin. Elevated levels can indicate insulin resistance, a major cause of type 2 diabetes.	<5 uIU/ml
Glucose (Fasting)	A blood glucose test is used to measure the amount of glucose (sugar) in the blood at the time of collection. If blood glucose levels remain high over a period of time, they can damage the eyes, kidneys, nerves, and blood vessels. High glucose levels indicate diabetes.	65–99 mg/dl
OGTT (Oral Glucose Tolerance Test)	A 1-hour and 2-hour glucose tolerance test can detect insulin resistance and new onset diabetes.	2hrs<140mg/dl

CARDIAC

Test	Definition	Optimal Results
CIMT (Carotid Intima-Media Thickness)	This test consists of an ultrasound of the carotid arteries and measures the thickness of the intima-media, a marker for atherosclerosis (plaque). It can detect accelerated disease processes and subclinical disease. It is a valuable tool for physicians to clarify cardiovascular risk of their patients, optimize prevention measures, and monitor the atherosclerotic process.	Negative
ABI (Ankle-Brachial Index)	A simple test that compares the blood pressure in your arm with the blood pressure in your ankle. Test detects peripheral artery disease and predicts cardiovascular mortality.	>0.90
AAA Screen (Abdominal Aortic Aneurysm Screen)	An ultrasound of the abdominal aorta to detect aneurysms. Recommended for men age 50 to 69 with at least one cardiovascular risk factor or African-Americans and all men 70 or older.	Negative
Cardiac Stress Testing	This test evaluates blood flow and determines if there are blockages interfering with the supply of blood and oxygen to your heart. It also provides valuable information regarding the fitness of your heart, blood vessels, and lungs. The test is performed on a treadmill or bike, while heart rate, blood pressure, and oxygen levels are monitored and recorded. This test can be completed in a clinic or hospital. Men age 45 and over should perform this test on a periodic basis.	Negative

Test	Definition	Optimal Results
Coronary Calcium Scoring	This test utilizes a CT Scan to assess coronary calcification and provides a score that is an anatomical test for total plaque burden. A positive score deserves additional evaluation and workup.	Zero

CARDIAC BLOOD TESTS

Test	Definition	Optimal Results
Homocysteine	High homocysteine levels are indicators of your risk for having heart disease, Alzheimer's disease, stroke, and vascular disease. These levels are strongly influenced by diet and genetics. It is recommended that men get tested if there is a family history of cardiovascular disease. Homocysteine levels should be checked every year.	<9 umol/l
Cardio C-Reactive Protein	Elevated C-reactive protein (CRP) indicates "silent inflammation": inflammation that is not linked to pain or infection. This blood test is used to assess risk for cardiovascular disease, aging, and all age-related diseases. CRP is typically tested at the same time a cholesterol screening is performed and is recommended as part of all routine blood chemistry screening.	<1.0 mg/l
Lp(a)-C	The lipoprotein (a)-C test provides additional information about your risk of developing heart disease. It is not included in routine blood work. This test is beneficial for men with existing vascular disease or who have a family history of coronary artery disease.	0–10 mg/dl
LDL-C	LDL (bad cholesterol) is obtained as part of your cholesterol panel and is also used to predict your risk of heart attack or stroke.	<70 mg/dl
HDL-C	HDL (good cholesterol) is obtained as part of your cholesterol panel. Low levels put you at risk for heart disease.	>50 mg/dl
Non-HDL-C	Total cholesterol minus HDL-C. May be used as a close surrogate to the ApoB. It is a better predictor of cardiovascular events than LDL-C.	<130mg/dl
Triglycerides	Triglycerides are the fat that is found in body fat tissue. Excess triglycerides are linked to coronary artery disease, diabetes, inflammation, cancer, and Alzheimer's disease. Triglycerides are measured along with cholesterol as part of a routine lipid panel test.	<100 mg/dl
ApoB	A blood test that is the single most significant and consistent lipid measurement to predict heart disease risk. A powerful marker of vascular disease and a better guide to the adequacy of therapy than any other lipid index. It represents the total burden of atherogenic lipoproteins.	<60
GFR (Glomerular Filtration Rate)	A blood test that assesses kidney function. It is a predictor of cardiovascular risk.	>60

Test	Definition	Optimal Results
F$_2$-isoprostanes	A blood test that predicts risk of coronary artery disease. A measure of oxidative stress.	>0.86 ng/mg
Vitamin D, 25-OH	Vitamin D deficiency increases heart attack risk in men.	50mg–80/dl
LpPLA2 (PLAC 2)	A blood test that is a cardiovascular-specific inflammatory enzyme involved in the formation of vulnerable rupture-prone plaque. It predicts risk for a stroke.	<80
Microalbumin-Creatine Ratio (ACR)	A simple and inexpensive urine test that is excellent for predicting cardiovascular disease risk.	<4.0µg/mg
Fibrinogen	A blood test that is a sensitive indicator of inflammation.	<450
Myeloperoxidase (MPO)	A blood test that is a strong indicator of a heart attack occurring over the next six months in seemingly healthy men.	<640
NT-proBNP	Valuable test for ventricular dysfunction—the "heart happy" test.	<125 pg/ml

GENETIC TESTING

Test	Definition	Optimal Results
TCF7L2	Genetic risk test for type 2 diabetes.	Negative
APO E Genotype	Genetic test used to guide therapy for CAD.	Results vary depending on genotype
KIF6	Genetic test that is a valuable predictor of risk for CAD.	Negative
LPA Gene Variant	Predicts CAD.	Negative
9P21	Predicts CAD.	Negative

HORMONES

Test	Definition	Optimal Results
Thyroid Panel	The thyroid gland is responsible for producing hormones that are essential for the body's metabolism. Thyroid hormones are analyzed through a blood sample. Symptoms such as fatigue, depression, cold intolerance, hair loss, headaches, fluid retention, unexplained weight gain or loss, anxiety, and panic attacks can be caused by thyroid abnormalities.	
Thyroid Stimulating Hormone (TSH)	TSH screening is used to diagnose and monitor treatment of thyroid disorders. TSH is released by the pituitary gland and stimulates the production of thyroid hormone. If there is an excessive amount of thyroid hormone, very little TSH is released and TSH levels fall. TSH levels help determine if you have hypothyroidism (production below normal) or hyperthyroidism (production above normal).	0.4–2.0 mu/l
Free T3	Used to help diagnose thyroid abnormalities. Free T3 is the unbound portion of T3 (triiodothyronine) that is responsible for its action in our bodies. Free T3 correlates most reliably with the clinical status of your thyroid and is responsible for controlling metabolism.	300–420 pg/dl 3.0–4.2 pg/ml
Free T4	Used to help diagnose thyroid abnormalities.	0.8–1.8 ng/dl

Test	Definition	Optimal Results
Total Testosterone	This test is used to measure the total amount of testosterone in the bloodstream.	700–1000 ng/dl
Free Testosterone	Free testosterone is the amount of unbound testosterone found in the blood. This is the form of testosterone that is available to all testosterone receptor sites located on cells throughout the body.	130–190 pg/ml
Dihydrotesterone (DHT)	Elevated DHT levels can cause hair loss and prostate enlargement. It is a breakdown product of testosterone metabolism.	25–75 ng/dl
Estradiol, High-Sensitivity	Produced by the adrenal glands and testes. Also another breakdown product of testosterone metabolism. Elevated estradiol can increase risk for stroke, breast enlargement, and prostate cancer. Men who are on testosterone replacement therapy should have their estradiol levels checked every 3 to 6 months.	10–40 pg/ml
ADRENAL		
Dehydroepiandrosterone (DHEA)	DHEA is a naturally occurring hormone produced in the adrenal glands, gonads, and brain. At age 30, DHEA levels begin to decrease naturally. Low DHEA levels are correlated to adrenal insufficiency, depression, obesity, lupus, Alzheimer's disease, bone density, cardiovascular disease, and chronic fatigue syndrome.	350–500 mcg/dl
Cortisol (Morning Level)	Cortisol is secreted by the adrenal gland and is known as the "stress" hormone because it is critical for survival. Excessive levels lead to increased storage of abdominal fat and heart disease.	<18 mcg/dl
PITUITARY		
Insulinlike Growth Factor 1, Somatomedin-C IGF-1 (indirect assay of growth hormone)	IGF-1 levels are directly related to growth hormone secretion from the pituitary gland. It is responsible for most of the physiological actions attributed to growth hormone.	200–320 ng/ml

Once you and your doctor have a clear understanding of your current health, you can follow the Life Plan knowing that you are taking care of yourself the best way possible. By adhering to the diet and exercise programs, you are ensuring that not only will you lose weight and gain muscle mass, but you will improve your heart health. If you follow the supplement program, you'll find that your energy levels will return. And if you carefully monitor your hormone levels, you'll find that in no time at all, you'll be looking and feeling younger. This extra vitality will carry over into every aspect of your life, from the bedroom to the boardroom. And you'll join me and the thousands of men just like you who have been enjoying a life full of great health and better sex by creating a stronger, leaner body.

Acknowledgments

I would first like to thank my wife, Annie, for all of her encouragement and support throughout this journey. Her contributions to this book have been nothing short of outstanding. I consider myself incredibly fortunate that she entered my life when she did, and she continues to provide me with the incentives I need to achieve optimal health.

Sarah Durand, Judith Curr, and the staff at Atria Books were tremendous to work with. They guided me, a first-time author, through the publishing maze in grand style, making it seem fun and exciting. My agent, Carol Mann, put together a phenomenal team with the folks at Atria and my publicist, Sandi Mendelson. I'd also like to thank Greta Blackburn for her support in this project and for introducing me to my writer, Pam Liflander.

Pam is not only a great person but a truly gifted writer who was able to help me tap into the essence of what I am all about, get my thoughts and beliefs on paper, and then organize and craft all of it into words that describe perfectly what men need to know to stay healthy and avoid getting old. She is not only my writer; she has become a dear friend.

Ever since I won the Body-*for*-LIFE Contest in 1998, I have wanted to write this book. Try as I might, I just couldn't find the words to make it happen. In 2006, I met Ann Castro and she became my voice, putting my thoughts to paper and outlining my ideas. Her creativity on the initial draft is reflected throughout my book. This book would have never happened without her help. I am honored to have her as a friend and consultant.

I also want to thank the many people who have been integral to my success and the success of my book. Ernie Baul, my previous trainer, was instrumental in helping me become a Grand Champion in the Body-*for*-LIFE contest. Rod Stanley, my current trainer and friend, has helped me reach a whole new level of fitness and physique; he also helped me craft the exercise and nutrition chapters of my book. Lauren Tancredi, my executive assistant, has played a huge role keeping me on task and sharing her honest opinions. Cicely Valenti helped to organize my research. Terry Goodlad, my photographer, did a fantastic job capturing me at my very best. Shane Gagne, my Pilates instructor, has turned a stiff old guy into a flexible youthful guy. Justin Won and Doris Hearrington, my Tae Kwon Do instructors, who continue to help me become a true martial artist. John Adams and the Cenegenics staff have been supportive from the very beginning. Last, I want to thank Dr. Brad Bale and Amy Doneen of the Bale/Doneen Method for all of their valuable information on preventing heart attacks and strokes.

Resources: www.DrLife.com

The DrLife.com website has up-to-date information to supplement this book. You'll find all of the forms necessary to create a journal recording your weight loss and exercise program. You'll also find the latest information and research on a variety of topics addressed in this book, including testosterone and growth hormone therapies to address deficiencies and the latest information on the telomere revolution. You will also find all of the supplement resources so that you can order the exact brands that I recommend.

You'll also find:

- One rep max calculator

- Skin fold testing for body composition

- Recommendations for protein bars and shakes

- Best water sources

- Calorie calculator and database

- Glycemic index

- Caloric index

- An updated listing of age management medicine physicians across the country

- And much more

References

On Hypnosis

1. Coué, Emile. *Self Mastery Through Conscious Autosuggestion.* London: Allen & Unwin, 1959.

2. Boyne, Gil. *Transforming Therapy: A New Approach to Hypnotherapy.* Glendale, Calif.: Westwood, 1989.

3. Simmerman, Tim. *Fundamentals of Hypnotism.* 1996. American Council of Hypnotist Examiners Approved.

On Testosterone

1. Annewieke, W. van den Beld, Frank H. de Jong, et al. Measures of bioavailable serum testosterone and estradiol and their relationships with muscle strength, bone density, and body composition in elderly men. *Journal of Clinical Endrocrinology & Metabolism.* Vol. 85, No. 9, 3276–82. 2000.

2. Bross, R., Javanbakht, M., and Bhasin, S. Anabolic interventions for aging-associated sarcopenia. *J Clin Endocrinol Metab.* Vol. 84, No. 10, 3420–30. 1999.

3. Tenover, J. S. Effects of testosterone supplementation in the aging male. *J Clin Endocrinol Metab.* 1992 Oct.; 75(4):1092–8.

4. Shalender, B., and Tenover, J. S. Age-Associated Sarcopenia—Issues in the use of testosterone as an anabolic agent in older men. *J Clin Endocrinol Metab.* Vol. 82, No. 6, 1659–60. 1997.

5. Urban, R. J., Bodenbrug, Y. H., et al. Testosterone administration to elderly men increases skeletal muscle strength and protein synthesis. *American Journal of Physiology.* 1995 Nov.; 269 (5 Pt 1):E820–6.

6. Snyder, P. The effects of testosterone treatment on body composition and metabolism in middle-aged obese men. *International Journal of Obesity and Related Metabolic Disorders.* 1992 Dec.; 16(12):991–7.

7. Snyder, P., Peachey, H., Hannoush, P., et al. Effect of testosterone treatment on bone mineral density in men over 65 years of age. *J Clin Endocrinol Metab.* Vol. 84, No. 6, 1966–72. 1999.

8. Marin, P., Holmang, S., Jonsson, L., Sjostrom, L., Kvist, H., et al. The effects of testosterone treatment on body composition and metabolism in middle-aged obese men. *Int J Obes Relat Metab Disord.* 1992 Dec.; 16(12):991–7.

9. Sundeep, Khosla, Melton, L. Joseph III, and Elizabeth, J. Relationship of serum sex steroid levels and bone turnover markers with bone mineral density in men and women: A key role for bioavailable estrogen. *J Clin Endocrinol Metab.* Vol. 83, No. 7, 2266–74. 1998.

10. Chute, G. Sex hormones and coronary artery disease. *American Journal of Medicine.* 1987 Nov.; 83(5):853–9.

11. Khaw, K. T., and Barrett-Connor, E. Lower endogenous androgens predict central adiposity in men. *Annals of Epidemiology.* 1992 Sep.; 2(5):675–82.

12. Khaw, K. T., and Barrett-Connor, E. Blood pressure and endogenous testosterone in men: an inverse relationship. *Journal of Hypertension.* 1988 Apr.; 6(4):329–32.

13. Marin, P., Krotkiewski, M., and Bjorntorp, P. Androgen treatment of middle-aged, obese men: effects on metabolism, muscle and adipose tissues. *European Journal of Medicine.* 1992 Oct.; 1(6):329–36.

14. Zmuda, J. M., Cauley, J. A., Kriska, A., Glynn, N. W., Gutai, J. P., and Kuller, L. H. Longitudinal relation between endogenous testosterone and cardiovascular disease risk factors in middle-aged men. A 13-year follow-up of former multiple risk factor intervention trial participants. *American Journal of Epidemiology.* 1997 Oct. 15; 146(8):609–17.

15. English, K. M., Mandour, O., Steeds, R. P., Diver, M. J., Jones, T. H., and Channer, K. S. Men with coronary artery disease have lower levels of androgens than men with normal coronary angiograms. *European Heart Journal.* 2000 Jun.; 21(11):890–4.

16. English, K. M., Steeds, R. P., Jones, T. H., Diver, M. J., and Channer, K. S. Low-dose transdermal testosterone therapy improves angina threshold in men with chronic stable angina: A randomized, double-blind, placebo-controlled study. *Circulation.* 2000 Oct. 17; 102(16):1906–11.

17. Wu, S. Z., and Weng, X. Z. Therapeutic effects of an androgenic preparation on myocardial ischemia and cardiac function in 62 elderly male coronary heart disease patients. *China Medical Journal (Engl).* 1993 Jun.; 106(6):415–8.

18. Webb, C. M., Adamson, D. L., de Zeigler, D., and Collins, P. Effect of acute testosterone on myocardial ischemia in men with coronary artery disease. *American Journal of Cardiology.* 1999 Feb. 1; 83(3):437–9, A9.

19. Muller, M. Endogenous sex hormones and cardiovascular disease in men. *J Clin Endocrinol Metab.* Vol. 88, No. 11, 5076–86. 2003.

20. Muller, M., Grobbee, D. E., den Tonkelaar, I., Lamberts, S. W., and van der Schouw, Y. T. Endogenous sex hormones and metabolic syndrome in aging men. *J Clin Endocrinol Metab.* 2005 May; 90(5):2618–23.

21. Rupprecht, R. Neuroactive steroids: Mechanisms of action and neuropsychopharmacological properties. *Psychoneuroendocrinology.* 2003 Feb.; 28(2):139–68.

22. Moffat, S. D., et al. Free testosterone and risk for Alzheimer disease in older men. *Neurology.* 2004 Jan. 27; 62(2):188–93.

23. Gouras, G. K., Xu, H., Gross, R. S., et al. Testosterone reduces neuronal secretion of Alzheimer's β-amyloid peptides. *Proceedings of the National Academy of Sciences of the United States of America.* 2000; 97:1202–5.

24. Papasozomenos, S. Ch., and Shanavas, A. Testosterone prevents the heat shock–induced overactivation of glycogen synthase kinase-3 beta but not of cyclin-dependent kinase 5 and c-Jun NH2-terminal kinase and concomitantly abolishes hyperphosphorylation of tau: Implications for Alzheimer's disease. *Proc Natl Acad Sci USA*. 2002 Feb. 5; 99(3):1140–5.

25. Gillett, M. J., Martins, R. N., Clarnette, R. M., Chubb, S. A., Bruce, D. G., and Yeap, B. B. Relationship between testosterone, sex hormone binding globulin and plasma amyloid beta peptide 40 in older men with subjective memory loss or dementia. *American Journal of Alzheimer's Disease*. 2003 Aug.; 5(4):267–9.

26. Tan, R. S., and Pu, S. J. A pilot study on the effects of testosterone in hypogonadal aging male patients with Alzheimer's disease. *Aging Male*. 2003 Mar.; 6(1):13–17.

27. Hogervorst, E., Combrinck, M., et al. Testosterone and gonadotropin levels in men with dementia. *Neuroendocrinology Letters*. 2003; 24(3–4):203–8.

28. Hogervorst, E., Bandelow, S., Combrinck, M., and Smith, A. D. Low free testosterone is an independent risk factor for Alzheimer's disease. *Experimental Gerontology*. 2004 Nov.–Dec.; 39(11–12):1633–9.

29. Paoletti, A. M., et al. Low androgenization index in elderly women and elderly men with Alzheimer's disease. *Neurology*. 2004 Jan. 27; 62(2):301–3.

30. Ramzi, R. Hajjar, Kaiser Fran E., and Morley, John E. Outcomes of long-term testosterone replacement in older hypogonadal males: A retrospective analysis. *J Clin Endocrinol Metab*. 1997 Vol. 82, No. 11, 3793–96.

31. Kwan, M., Greenleaf, W. J., Mann, J., Crapo, L., and Davidson, J. M. The nature of androgen action on male sexuality: A combined laboratory-self-report study on hypogonadal men. *J Clin Endocrinol Metab*. 1983 Vol. 57, 557–62.

32. Skakkebaek, N. E., Bancroft, J., Davidson, D. W., and Warner, P. Androgen replacement with oral testosterone undecenoate in hypogonadal men: A double blind controlled study. *Clinical Endocrinology (Oxf)*. 1981 Jan.; 14:49–61.

33. O'Carroll, R., and Bancroft, J. Testosterone therapy for low sexual interest and erectile dysfunction in men: A controlled study. *British Journal of Psychiatry*. 1984 Aug.; 145:146–51.

34. Ebert, T., Jockenhovel, F., Morales, A., et al. The current status of therapy for symptomatic late-onset hypogonadism with transdermal testosterone gel. *European Urology*. 2005 Feb.; 47(2):137–46.

35. Carani, C., Zini, D., Baldini, A., et al. Effects of androgen treatment in impotent men with normal and low levels of free testosterone. *Archives of Sexual Behavior*. 1990 Jun.; 19(3):223–34.

36. Jain, J. Effect of exogenous testosterone on prostate volume, serum and semen prostate specific antigen levels in healthy young men. *Journal of Urology*. 1998 Feb.; 159(2):441–3.

37. Cooper, C. S., Perry, P. J., Sparks, et al. Effect of exogenous testosterone on prostate volume, serum and semen prostate specific antigen levels in healthy young men. *J Urol*. 1998 Feb.; 159(2):441–3.

38. Margolese, H. C. The male menopause and mood: Testosterone decline and depression in the aging male—is there a link? *Journal of Geriatric Psychiatry and Neurology*. 2000 Summer; 13(2):93–101.

39. Morley, J. E. Testosterone replacement and the physiologic aspects of aging in men. *Mayo Clinic Proceedings*. 2000 Jan.; 75 Suppl:S83–7.

40. Basaria, Shehzad, Wahlstrom, Justin T., and Dobs, Adrian S. Anabolic-androgenic steroid therapy in the treatment of chronic diseases. *J Clin Endocrinol Metab.* Vol. 86, No. 11, 5108–17. 2001.

41. Hoffman, M. A., DeWolf, W. C., and Morgentaler, A. Is low serum free testosterone a marker for high grade prostate cancer? *J Urol.* 2000 Mar.; 163(3):824–7.

42. Asbell, S. O., Raimane, K. C., Montesano, A. T., Zeitzer, K. L., Asbell, M. D., and Vijayakumar, S. Prostate-specific antigen and androgens in African-American and white normal subjects and prostate cancer patients. *Journal of the National Medical Association.* 2000 Sep.; 92(9):445–9.

43. Rhoden, E. L., and Morgentaler, A. Risks of testosterone-replacement therapy and recommendations for monitoring. *New England Journal of Medicine.* 2004 Jan. 29; 350(5):482–92.

44. Carter, H. B., et al. Longitudinal evaluation of serum androgen levels in men with and without prostate cancer. *Prostate.* 1995 Jul.; 27(1):25–31.

45. Conway, H. J. Randomized clinical trial of testosterone replacement therapy in hypogonadal men. *International Journal of Andrology.* 1988 Aug.; 11(4):247–64.

46. Pugh, Peter, Jones, T. Hugh, and Channer, Kevin. Acute haemodynamic effects of testosterone in men with chronic heart failure. *Eur Heart J.* 2003, 24, 909–15.

47. Caminiti, Giuseppe, Volterrani, Maurizio, et al. Effect of long-acting testosterone treatment on function exercise capacity, skeletal muscle performance, insulin resistance, and baroreflex sensitivity in elderly patients with chronic heart failure: A double-blind, placebo controlled, randomized study. *J Am Coll. Cardiol.* 2009; 54:919–27.

48. Malkin, Chris J., et al. Testosterone therapy in men with moderate severity heart failure: a double-blind randomized placebo controlled trial. *Eur Heart J.* 2006, 24, 54–64.

49. Hyde, Zoe, et al. Low free testosterone predicts frailty in older men: The health in men study. *J Clin Endocrinol Metab.* April 21, 2001 (95) 7, 3165–72.

50. Menke, Andy, et al. Sex steroid hormone concentrations and risk of death in US men. *Am J Epidemiol.* 2009 (171) 5, 583–92.

51. Srinivas-Shankar, Upendram. Effects of testosterone on muscle strength, physical function, body composition and quality of life in intermediate-frail and frail elderly men: A randomized, double-blind, placebo-controlled study. *J Clin Endocrinol Metab.* 2010 (95) 2, 639–50.

52. Sattler, F. R., et al. Testosterone and growth hormone improve body composition and muscle performance in older men. *J Clin Endocrinol Metab.* 2009 (94) 6, 1991–2001.

53. Maggio, Marcello, et al. Relationship between low levels of anabolic hormones and 6-year mortality rate in older men. *Archives of Internal Medicine.* 2007 (167) 20, 2249–54.

54. Wu, Frederick, C. W., et al. Identification of late-onset hypogonadism in middle-aged and elderly men. *N Engl J Med.* 2010 (363):123–35.

On Growth Hormone

1. Society for Endocrinology, Practice and Policy, Growth Hormone, http://www.endocrinology.org/policy/docs/gh.html.

2. Fowelin, J., Attrall, S., Lager, I., and Bengtsson, B.-Å. Effects of treatment with recombinant human growth hormone on insulin sensitivity and glucose metabolism in adults with growth hormone deficiency. *Metabolism.* 1993, 42, 1443–7.

3. Johansson, J.-Q., Landin, K., Tengboru, L., Rosén, T., and Bengtsson, B.-Å. High fibrinogen and plasminogen activator inhibitor activity in growth hormone deficient adults. *Arteriosclerosis, Thrombosis, and Vascular Biology.* 1994, 14, 434–7.

4. Markussis, V., Beshyah, S. A., Fischer, C., Sharp, P., Nicolaides, A. N., and Johnson, D. G. Detection of premature atherosclerosis by high resolution ultrasonography in symptom-free hypopituitary adults. *Lancet.* 1992, 340, 1188–92.

5. Capaldo, B., Patti, L., Oliverio, U., Longobardi, S., Pardo, F., Vitali, F., Fazio, S., di Reller, F., Bindi, B., Lombardi, G., and Sacca, L. Increased arterial intimi-media thickness in childhood onset growth hormone deficiency. *J Clin Endocrinol Metab.* 1997, 82, 1378–81.

6. Rosén, T., and Bengtsson, B.-Å. Premature mortality due to cardiovascular disease in hypopituitarism. *Lancet.* 1990, 336, 285–8.

7. Bülow, B., Hacrmar, L., Mikoczy, Z., Nordström, C. H., and Erfurth, E. M. Increased cerebrovascular mortality in patient with hypopituitarism. *Clinical Endocrinology.* 1997, 46, 75–81.

8. American Association of Clinical Endocrinologist Medical Guidelines for Clinical Practice for Growth Hormone Use in Growth Hormone Deficient Adults and Transition Patients—October 2009 Update. *Endocrine Practice.* 2009; 15(2):1.

9. Murray, R., Bidlingmaier, M., Strasburger, C., and Shalet, S. The diagnosis of partial growth hormone deficiency in adults with a putative insult to the hypothalamo-pituitary axis. *J Clin Endocrinol Metab.* 2007. 92(5):1705–9.

10. Consensus Statement. Consensus guidelines for the diagnosis and treatment of adults with GH deficiency II: A statement of the GH Research Society in association with the European Society for Pediatric Endocrinology, Lawson Wilkins Society, European Society of Endocrinology, Japan Endocrine Society, and Endocrine Society of Australia. *European Journal of Endocrinology.* 2007. 157: 695–700.

11. Murray, R. D., and Shalet, S. M. Insulin sensitivity is impaired in adults with varying degrees of GH deficiency. *Clin Endocrinol.* 2005 Feb.; 62(2):182–8.

12. Murray R. D., Adams, J. E., and Shalet, S. M. Adults with partial growth hormone deficiency have an adverse body composition. *J Clin Endocrinol Metab.* 2004 Apr.; 89(4):1586–91.

13. Colao, A., Cerbone, G., Pivonello, R., Aimaretti, G., Loche, S., Di Somma, C., Faggiano, A., Corneli, G., Ghigo, E., and Lombardi, G. The growth hormone (GH) response to the arginine plus GH-releasing hormone test is correlated to the severity of lipid profile abnormalities in adult patients with GH deficiency. *J Clin Endocrinol Metab.* 1999 Apr.; 84(4):1277–82.

14. Colao, A., Di Somma, C., Spiezia, S., Rota, F., Pivonello, R., Savastano, S., and Lombardi, G. The natural history of partial growth hormone deficiency in adults: A prospective study on the cardiovascular risk and atherosclerosis. *J Clin Endocrinol Metab.* 2001 Jun.; 91(6):2191–200.

15. Pandian, Rai, and Nakamoto, Jon M. Rational use of the laboratory for childhood and adult growth hormone deficiency. *Clin Lab Med.* 2004 Mar.; 24(1):141–74.

16. Vestergaard, P., and Hoeck, H. C. Reproducibility of growth hormone and cortisol responses to the insulin tolerance test and the short ACTH test in normal adults. *Horm Metab Res.* 1997 Mar.; 29(3):106–10.

17. Hoeck, H. C. Test of growth hormone secretion in adults: Poor reproducibility of the insulin tolerance test. *Eur J Endocrinol.* 1995 Sep.; 133(3):305–12.

18. Biller, B. Sensitivity and specificity of six tests for the diagnosis of adult GH deficiency. *J Clin Endocrinol Metab.* 2002 May; 87(5):2067–79.

19. Hoeck, H. C. Diagnosis of growth hormone (GH) deficiency in adults with hypothalamic-pituitary disorders: Comparison of test results using pyridostigmine plus GH-releasing hormone (GHRH), clonidine plus GHRH, and insulin-induced hypoglycemia as GH secretagogues. *J Clin Endocrinol Metab.* 2000 Apr.; 85(4):1467–72.

20. Boquete, H. R. Evaluation of diagnostic accuracy of insulin-like growth factor (IGF)-I and IGF-binding protein-3 in growth hormone-deficient children and adults using ROC plot analysis. *J Clin Endocrinol Metab.* 2003 Oct.; 88(10):4702–8.

21. Bonert, V. S. Body mass index determines evoked growth hormone (GH) responsiveness in normal healthy male subjects: Diagnostic caveat for adult GH deficiency. *J Clin Endocrinol Metab.* 2004 Jul.; 89(7):3397–3401.

22. Hartman, M. L., et al. Which patients do not require a GH stimulation test for the diagnosis of adult GH deficiency? *J Clin Endocrinol Metab.* 2002 Feb.; 87(2):477–85.

23. Carroll, et al. Growth hormone deficiency in adulthood and the effects of growth hormone replacement: A review. Growth Hormone Research Society Scientific Committee. *J Clin Endocrinol Metab.* 1998 Feb.; 83(2):382–95.

24. Franco, C. Growth hormone treatment reduces abdominal visceral fat in postmenopausal women with abdominal obesity: A 12-month placebo-controlled trial. *J Clin Endocrinol Metab.* 2005 Mar.; 90(3):1466–74.

25. Albert, S. Low-dose recombinant human growth hormone as adjuvant therapy to lifestyle modifications in the management of obesity. *J Clin Endocrinol Metab.* 2004 Feb.; 89(2).

26. Johannsson, G. Growth hormone treatment of abdominally obese men reduces abdominal fat mass, improves glucose and lipoprotein metabolism, and reduces diastolic blood pressure. *J Clin Endocrinol Metab.* 1997 Mar.; 82(3):725–26.

27. http://www.ghresearchsociety.org/bin/Default.asp.

28. Larsen, Kronnenberg, Melmed, and Polonsky (eds). *Williams Textbook of Endocrinology.* Saunders, 2003, Tenth Edition, Chapter 8, authored by Shlomo Melmed and David Kleinberg, summarizes adult somatotropin deficiency in Table 8–20, p. 226, and they point out that IGF-1 levels may be "low or normal" in adult deficiency states.

29. Colao, A., et al. The national history of partial growth hormone deficiency in adults: A prospective study on cardiovascular risk and atheroscelerosis. *J Clin Endocrinol Metabol.* 91(6):2191–2200.

30. Drake, W. M. Optimizing growth hormone therapy in adults and children. *Endocr Rev.* 2001 Aug. 1; 22(4):425–50.

31. Mukherjee, A. Seeking the optimal target range for insulin-like growth factor I during the treatment of adult growth hormone disorders. *J Clin Endocrinol Metab.* 2003 Dec.; 88(12):5865–70.

32. Roubenof, R. Cytokines, insulin-like growth factor-1, sarcopenia, and mortality in very old community-dwelling men and women: The Framingham Heart Study. *Am J Med.* 2003 Oct. 15; 115(6):429–35.

33. Cappola, A. Insulin-like growth factor I and interleukin-6 contribute synergistically to disability and mortality in older women. *J Clin Endocrinol Metab.* 2003 May; 88(5):2019–25.

34. Laughlin, G. A., et al. The prospective association of serum insulin-like growth factor I (IGF-I) and IGF-binding protein-1 levels with all cause and cardiovascular disease mortality in older adults: The Rancho Bernardo Study. *J Clin Endocrinol Metab.* 2004 Jan.; 89(1):114–20.

35. Gelato, M. Aging and immune function: A possible role for growth hormone. *Hormone Research.* 1996; 45:46–49.

36. Toogood, A. A., et al. Beyond the somatopause: Growth hormone deficiency in adults over the age of 60 years. *J Clin Endocrinol Metab.* 1996 Feb; 81(2):460–65.

37. Young, A. Muscle function in old age. *New Issue Neuroscience.* 1998; I:141–56.

38. Skeleton, D. A., et al. Strength, power & related functional ability of healthy people aged 60–89 years. *Aging People.* 1994; 23:371–77.

39. Bohannon, R. W. Comfortable and maximum walking speed of adults aged 20–79 years: Reference values and determinants. *Age Ageing.* 1997; 26:15–19.

40. O'Connor: Ph.D. thesis, Dublin, 1998.

41. Vahl, N., et al. Abdominal adiposity and physical fitness are major determinants of age associated decline in stimulated growth hormone secretion in healthy adults. *J Clin Endocrinol Metab.* 1996 Jun; 81(6): 2209–15.

42. Savine, R., and Sonksen, P. Growth hormone—hormone replacement for somatopause. *Horm Res.* 2000; 53(Suppl 3):37–41.

43. Conti, E., et al. Insulin-like growth factor-1 as a vascular protective factor. *Circulation.* 2004; 110:2260–65.

44. Denti, L., et al. Insulin-like growth factor 1 as a predictor of ischemic stroke outcome in the elderly. *Am J Med.* 2004 Sep.; 117(5):312–17.

45. Juul, A., et al. Low serum insulin-like growth factor-1 is associated with increased risk of ischemic heart disease: A population-based case-control study. *Circulation.* 2002; 106:939–44.

46. Vasan, R. S., et al. Serum insulin-like growth factor-1 and risk for heart failure in elderly individuals without a previous myocardial infarction: The Framingham Heart Study. *Ann Intern Med.* 2003; 139:642–48.

47. Molitch, Mark E., et al. Evaluation and treatment of AGHD: An Endocrine Society Clinical Practice Guideline. *J Clinical Endocrinol Metab.* 2006; 91(5):1621–34.

48. Consensus guideline for the diagnosis and treatment of adults with growth hormone deficiency II. *Eur J Endrocrinol.* 2007 Dec.; 157(6):695–700.

49. Melmed, S. Supplemental growth hormone in healthy adults: The endocrinologist's responsibility. *Nature Clinical Practice.* 2006; 2:119.

50. Critical evaluation of the safety of recombinant human growth hormone administration: Statement from the Growth Hormone Research Society. *J Clin Endocrinol Metab.* 2001; 86(5):1868–70.

51. Bjorntorp, P. "Portal" adipose tissue as a generator of risk factors for cardiovascular disease and diabetes. *Arteriosclerosis.* 1990; 10:493–96.

52. Veldhuis, J. D. Neuroendocrine control of pulsatile growth hormone release in the human: Relationship with gender. *Growth Hormone IGF-1 Res 8 (Suppl B).* 1998; 49–59.

53. Vahl, N., et al. Abdominal adiposity rather than age and sex predicts mass and regularity of GH secretion in healthy adults. *Am J Physiol.* 1997; 272:E1108–16.

54. Pasarica, M., et al. Effect of growth hormone on body composition and visceral adiposity in middle-aged men with visceral obesity. *J Clin Endocrinol Metab.* 2007 Nov; 9211:4265–70.

55. Beauregard, C., et al. Growth hormone decreases visceral fat and improves cardiovascular risk markers in women with hypopituitarism: A randomized, placebo-controlled study. *J Clin Endocrinol Metab.* First published ahead of print April 1, 2008 as doi:10.1210/jc.2007–71.

56. Simpson, H., et al. Growth hormone replacement therapy for adults: Into the new millennium. *Growth Horm IGF Res.* 2002; 12:1–33.

57. De Boer, H., et al. Clinical aspects of growth hormone deficiency in adults. *Endocr Rev.* 1995; 16:63–86.

58. Bengtsson, B.-Å., et al. Treatment of adults with growth hormone deficiency: Results of a 13-month placebo controlled cross over study. *Clin Endocrinol (Oxf).* 1993; 76:309–17.

59. Snel, Y. E., et al. Magnetic resonance image-assessed adipose tissue and serum lipid and insulin concentrations in growth hormone deficient adults: Effects of growth hormone replacement. *Arterioscler Thromb Vasc Biol.* 1995; 15:1543–48.

60. Hartman, M., et al. Growth hormone replacement therapy in adults with growth hormone deficiency improves maximal oxygen consumption independently of dosing regimen or physical activity. *J Clin Endocrinol Metab.* 2008 Jan.; 93(1):125–30.

61. Kwan, A., and Hartman, M. IGF-1-1 measurements in the diagnosis of adult growth hormone deficiency. *Pituitary.* 2007; 10(2):151–57.

62. Clemmons, D. R., and Underwood, L. E. Nutritional regulation of IGF-1-1 and IGF-1 binding proteins. *Annu Rev Nutr.* 1991; 11:393–412.

63. Hartman, M. L. Physiological regulators of growth hormone secretion. In Juul, A., and Jorgensen, J. O. L. (eds). *Growth Hormone in Adults,* 2nd ed. Cambridge: Cambridge University Press, 2000, pp. 3–53.

64. Baker, H. W., et al. Arginine-infusion test for growth-hormone secretion. *Lancet.* 1970; 2(7684):1193.

65. Juul, A. Serum levels of insulin-like growth factor I and its binding proteins in health and disease. *Growth Horm IGF-1 Res.* 2003; 13:113–70.

66. Larsson, S. C., et al. Association of diet with serum insulin-like growth factor I in middle aged and elderly men. *Am J Clin Nutr.* 2005; 81:1163–67.

67. Clasey, J. L., et al. Abdominal visceral fat and fasting insulin are important predictors of 24-hr GH release independent of age, gender, and other physiological factors. *J Clin Endocrinol Metab.* 2001 Aug.; 86(8):3845–52.

68. Rasmussen, M. H., et al. Massive weight loss restores 24-hr growth hormone release profiles and serum insulin-like growth factor-1 levels in obese subjects. *J Clin Endocrinol Metab.* 1995 Apr; 80(4):1407–15.

69. Giustina, A., and Veldhuis, J. D. Pathophysiology of the neuroregulation of growth hormone secretion in experimental animals and the human. *Endocrin Review.* 1998; 19(6):717–97.

70. Felsing, N. E., et al. Effect of low and high intensity exercise on circulating growth hormone in men. *J Clin Endocrinol Metab.* 1992 Jul; 75(1):157–62.

71. Weltman, A., et al. Endurance training amplifies the pulsatile release of growth hormone: Effects of training intensity. *J Appl Physiol.* 1992; 72(6):2188–96.

72. Weltman, A., et al. Relationship between age, percentage body fat, fitness and 24-hour growth hormone release in healthy young adults: Effect of gender. *J Clin Endocrinol Metab.* 1994 Mar; 78(3):543–48.

73. Vahl, N., et al. Abdominal adiposity and physical fitness are major determinants of the age associated decline in stimulated GH secretion in healthy adults. *J Clin Endocrinol Metab.* 1996 Jun; 81(6):2209–15.

74. Yuen, K., et al. Is lack of recombinant growth hormone (GH)-releasing hormone in the United States a setback or time to consider glucagon testing for adult GH deficiency? *J Clin Endocrinol Metab.* 2009; 94:2702–7.

75. Holt, R. Growth hormone: A potential treatment option in diabetes? *Diabetic Voice.* Jul. 2003, Vol. 48, Issue 2.

76. Cauter, E., et al. Age-related changes in slow wave sleep and REM sleep and relationship with growth hormone and cortisol levels in healthy men. *JAMA.* Aug. 16, 2000. 284, No. 7, 861–67.

77. Van Bunderen, Christa C., et al. The association of serum insulin-like growth factor-I with mortality, cardiovascular disease, and cancer in the elderly: A population-based study. *J Clin Endocrinol Metab.* 2010 Oct; 95(9):4449–54.

78. Popovic, Vera, et al. Serum insulin-like growth factor I (IGF-I), IGF-binding proteins 2 and 3 and the risk for development of malignancies in adults with growth hormone (GH) deficiency treated with GH: Data from KIMS (Pfizer International Metabolic Database). *J Clin Endocrinol Metab.* 2010 (Online).

79. Meinhardt, Udo, M. D., et al. The effects of growth hormone on body composition and physical performance in recreational athletes: A randomized trial. *Annals of Internal Medicine.* May 4, 2010 (152) 9, 568–77.

80. Movérare-Skrtic, S., et al. Serum insulin-like growth factor-I concentration is associated with leukocyte telomere length in a population-based cohort of elderly men. *J Clin Endocrinol Metab.* 2009 Dec; 94(12):5078–84.

81. Makimura, H., et al. Reduced growth hormone secretion is associated with increased carotid intima-media thickness in obesity. *J Clin Endocrinol Metab.* 2009 Dec; 94(12):5131–38.

82. Colao, A., et al. Growth hormone treatment on atherosclerosis: Results of a 5-year open, prospective, controlled study in male patients with severe growth hormone deficiency. *J Clin Endocrinol Metab.* 2008 Sep; 93(9):3416–24.

83. Colao, A., et al. The natural history of partial growth hormone deficiency in adults: A prospective study on cardiovascular risk and atherosclerosis. *J Clin Endocrinol Metab.* 2006 Jun; 91(6):2191–2200.

84. Colao, A., et al. Short-term effects of growth hormone (GH) treatment or deprivation on cardiovascular risk parameters and intima-media thickness at carotid arteries in patients with severe GH deficiency. *J Clin Endocrinol Metab.* 2005 Apr; 90(4):2056–62.

85. Cittadini, Antonio, et al. Growth hormone deficiency in patients with chronic heart failure and beneficial effects of its correction. *J Clin Endocrinol Metab.* 2009 Sep; 94(9):3329–36.

86. Fazio, Sarfino, et al. Effects of growth hormone on exercise capacity and cardiopulmonary performance in patients with chronic heart failure. *J Clin Endocrinol Metab.* 2007 Nov; 92(11):4218–23.

87. Le Corvoisier, Philippe, et al. Cardiac effects of growth hormone treatment in chronic heart failure: A meta-analysis. *J Clin Endocrinol Metab.* 2007 Jan; 92(1):180–85.

88. Sattler, F. R., et al. Testosterone and growth hormone improve body composition and muscle performance in older men. *J Clin Endocrinol Metab.* 2009 Jun; 94(6):1991–2001.

89. Brugts, M. P., et al. Low circulating insulin-like growth factor I bioactivity in elderly men is associated with increased mortality. *J Clin Endocrinol Metab.* 2008 Jun; 93(7):2515–22.

90. Savastano, S., et al. Growth hormone treatment prevents loss of lean mass after bariatric surgery in morbidly obese patients: Results of a pilot, open, prospective randomized controlled study. *J Clin Endocrinol Metab.* 2009 Mar; 94(3):817–26.

Index

therapy with, 287–88, 290–91, 312
hunger, 84, 256–57
hypnosis, 260–70
    entering hypnotic state and, 261–62
    stress and, 262, 267–68
    success with, 264–65

immunity, 7, 34, 117, 224, 267
    and Life Plan for Healthy Eating rules, 55, 58–60
    medical breakthroughs and, 311, 314
    nutraceuticals and, 301–2
insulin, 18, 22, 32–37, 50, 282, 290–91, 293, 295, 320
    exercise and, 34–35, 44, 117, 168–69, 225
    Life Plan Diets and, 70, 73–74
    and Life Plan for Healthy Eating rules, 51–52, 57, 61–64
    Metabolic Syndrome and, 33–36
    nutrition and, 32, 34–36
intensity, 177

jumps:
    advanced box, 208
    crunch to, pull-ups, 181, 194–95, 218
    squat, 182–83, 209

kale soup, "Not So Portuguese," 76, 80, 88, 91, 96, 98, 106
Kegels, 283–84
kick backs, 180, 216
knee grabs, walking, 149

lat stretch, 136
legs, workouts and, 133–34, 144, 148, 153, 157–60, 162, 165, 172, 175, 179–80, 182, 194, 202–9, 213, 218, 220, 238
legumes, 55, 61, 299
    Life Plan Diets and, 74, 81–82, 88–89, 91–99, 101–3, 106
Lewin, Larry L., 304

Life Plan:
    evaluating progress in, 257–58
    forever, 109–10
Life Plan Diets, *see* Basic Health Diet; Fat-Burning Diet; Heart Health Diet
Life Plan for Healthy Eating:
    and nutrition, 31–68
    rules for, 51–68
lifestyle, 20–21, 25, 28, 48
    exercise and, 20, 224, 249
    hormones and, 21, 50, 282
lifts, dead, 156, 180, 205, 292
long slow distance training (LSD), 237–38
low-fat diets, 5, 7, 19, 26, 59–60, 282–83
lunches, 53, 67, 106–7
lunges:
    barbell, 180, 204
    to curl, 213
    side, 152
    walking, overhead press, 218–19
lung function, 224, 238
lycopene, 298, 302–3

macronutrient ratios, 51, 54–66
margarine, 58–59
martial arts, 10, 149, 151–52
max effort zone, 235
meals:
    frequency of, 51–54, 67, 74, 84, 256
    Life Plan Diets and, 54, 74, 76–103
    and Life Plan for Healthy Eating rules, 51–54, 67
    skipping of, 52–53
    times for, 43–44, 52
meats, 31, 42–43
    Life Plan Diets and, 73, 75, 77, 79, 84–85, 98, 101, 106
    and Life Plan for Healthy Eating rules, 55, 57, 59, 62–63
    preparation of, 75
medical breakthroughs, 307–14
    in genetic testing and therapy,

307–11
    in stem cell banking and therapy, 307, 311–13
    in telomeres, 307, 313–14
medications, 19–20, 25, 41, 114–16, 169–70, 173, 316, 320
    health-care system and, 16–17
    nutraceuticals and, 301–2, 304
    sex and, 114, 284
Medina, Rafael, 72
melatonin, 284–85, 297
metabolic equivalents (METs), 225–31, 235–37
Metabolic Syndrome, 26, 169–70
    components of, 28, 33–34
    hormones and, 28, 33–36, 275, 289–90
    nutrition and, 32–33
metabolism, 19, 32, 37, 40–43, 45, 117–18, 296, 310, 315, 317
    energy and, 42–43
    exercise and, 42–43, 121, 123, 168, 221, 224–25, 239
    hormones and, 33–34, 42, 322–23
    and Life Plan for Healthy Eating rules, 51–53, 57, 64–66
milk, 44, 55, 62, 300–301, 303
    Life Plan Diets and, 70–72, 76, 79, 83, 85
milk thistle, 298, 303
minerals, 74, 295–98
    difference between vitamins and, 297
    supplementing with, 295, 297–98, 303–6
mitochondria, 27, 118–19, 169
muscle, 4, 6–9, 15, 19–22, 40, 42, 44, 49, 66–67, 72, 109, 114–19, 122, 266, 318–19
    exercise and, 27, 116–19, 121, 123–25, 129–31, 135–42, 149–51, 155, 167–79, 181, 183–222, 224, 233–34, 238, 246–47, 253, 255, 257, 283–84, 296–97
    hormones and, 27, 34–37, 275–76, 278–79, 281–83, 287–90